The Ultimate OSCE Histories Guide

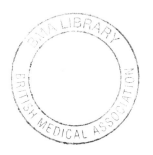

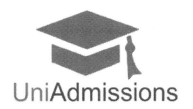

UniAdmissions

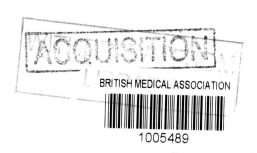

ISBN 978-1-912557-01-1

Published by RAR Medical Services Limited
www.uniadmissions.co.uk
info@uniadmissions.co.uk
Tel: 0208 068 0438

ABOUT THE AUTHORS

Miguel is a **5th year medical student** at King's College London, currently ranked in the **top one percent** of his cohort. He completed an intercalated BSc in Anatomy, Developmental and Human Biology, graduating with first class honours. His motivation for writing this book was to impart knowledge that he has acquired to help fellow students excel in their OSCEs.

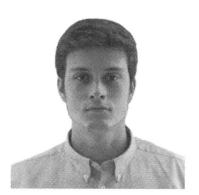

Miguel is passionate about a career in surgery and has been involved in numerous research projects, conferences and national audits. Through his involvement with different organisations, he has taught hundreds of individuals including young offenders from disadvantaged backgrounds and other medical students. In his free time, Miguel enjoys kickboxing, which he has practiced since the age of 5.

Aayushi graduated from Imperial College London School of Medicine with a **Distinction in Clinical Sciences** after completing her undergraduate degree in Natural Sciences from the University of Cambridge (Neuroscience (BA) Hons.). She was amongst the **top ten students** in her final year OSCEs and was awarded multiple distinctions throughout medical school. She completed a prestigious Academic Foundation Programme in 2017 and has presented original research on childhood asthma internationally in Sydney and Milan.

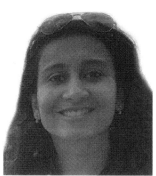

She has a keen interest in teaching and a desire to impart knowledge to the next generation of doctors to help them be the very best they can. In her free time, Aayushi enjoys playing the ukulele and badminton.

Rohan is the **Director of Operations** at *UniAdmissions* and is responsible for its technical and commercial arms. He graduated from Gonville and Caius College, Cambridge and is a qualified doctor. Over the last five years, he has tutored hundreds of successful Oxbridge and Medical applicants. He has also authored twenty books on admissions tests and interviews.

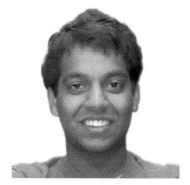

Rohan has taught physiology to undergraduates and interviewed medical school applicants for Cambridge. He has published research on bone physiology and writes education articles for the Independent and Huffington Post. In his spare time, Rohan enjoys playing the piano and table tennis.

The Ultimate OSCE Histories Guide

Miguel Sequeira Campos
Aayushi Sen
Rohan Agarwal

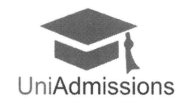

UniAdmissions

PREFACE

Thinking about it, OSCEs are a scary, scary idea. After years of practicing and perfecting sitting written exams, you're faced with going into a room, facing an unknown scenario with a stranger and an examiner scrutinising your every move, every question, every answer. It's enough terrify anyone. And then the "What if?.." scenarios: What if I don't get the diagnosis? What if I freeze? What if I forget to ask something? What if, what if, what if...

I remember my first OSCE at Imperial College Medical School. To help students prepare for their first OSCEs, the medical school release the stations that will be examined 24 hours prior to test day. Normally these are straightforward e.g. "Chest Pain" or "Polyuria". However, in my year, this list contained an unusual station: "Palpation history". Everyone panicked and speculated about what this could possibly be. Palpitations perhaps? Or a history about something the patient palpated on themselves? A peripheral vascular exam?! Most people favoured the former and persistently asked probing questions about strange feelings in the chest and cardiac risk factors (not believing the patient's insistence that they had no such thing!).

The station turned out to have been mislabelled – it was actually an asthma attack. The students that passed listened to the symptoms given to them and systematically approached it to realise that although there were no palpitations (best to make sure!), there was shortness of breath and wheeze.

There are a million "What if" scenarios which could happen, but you can handle them all if you keep your cool and have a systematic approach. OSCEs are not malevolent. They aren't there to trip you up, just make sure you are rational, systematic and safe.

Remember, at a medical school level - they are a test of competence rather than excellence. This doesn't change the fact that OSCEs can be scary and different to what you're used to, but if you prepare the right way you will be able to do yourself justice. It's all about practice. Practice histories and examinations over and over with as many patients, friends and family members as will allow you to. I hope this book gives you that system and practice crucial to doing well in your upcoming OSCEs and I wish you all the best of luck!

Dr. Aayushi Sen

The purpose of this book is to teach medical students the process of taking a *focused* history – the foundation of medical practice and something that often proves daunting for those transitioning from their pre-clinical to clinical studies.

Although a firm grasp of medical theory is the most important component of a good history, it is possible to score highly in an OSCE without extensive knowledge. However, this can only be achieved with solid frameworks, breaking down series of questions into logical blocks – making it easy to structure and, to an extent, control your interaction with your patient (or, in the context of an OSCE, actor).

There are resources currently on the market but none quite like this. This book provides solid frameworks you can apply to any scenario, even ones you have not previously encountered. It will take you through common presenting complaints, step-by-step, highlighting important questions to ask and providing a differential diagnosis with respective findings, suggested investigations and management plans. There are over 100 sample histories for you to practice accompanied by comprehensive mark schemes. I hope that you find this book useful in your OSCE preparation and I welcome all feedback to help make this an increasingly useful resource. I am also happy to inform you that, as a way of giving back, I will be donating the entirety of my royalties to a medical charity.

Finally, it would be remiss of me not to mention the importance of regularly clerking patients and actively seeking learning opportunities during your time in a healthcare setting. Our desire to care for patients is (or should be) the reason we are all at medical school and if you are confident in your ability to communicate with patients, doing so in the context of an assessment should be no more challenging. Good luck!

Miguel Barros de Sequeira Campos

Acknowledgements

Gostaria de dedicar este livro aos meus pais, Isabel e Miguel, e à minha irmã Marta, que me apoiam incondicionalmente e a quem eu devo tanto.

I would like to dedicate this book to my parents, Isabel and Miguel, and my sister Marta, who support me unconditionally and to whom I owe so much.

Thank you to Ms. Despoina Nikolaidi for proofreading the penultimate version of this manuscript, providing valuable advice and a significant re-structuring. Thank you to Rohan for his support and guidance in realising the vision I had for this book.

Miguel

Thanks to my teachers. The good ones who imparted both knowledge and wisdom; the great ones who taught me what it meant to be a good teacher. I hope this book does them proud, and does you some good. Best of luck!

Aayushi

CONTENTS

INTRODUCTION

This introductory chapter aims to explain the purpose of an OSCE and then goes into a little more depth about the history-taking component.

What is an OSCE?

An OSCE, or Organised Structured Clinical Examination, is a practical exam consisting of a set of stations aiming to assess your ability to perform in a clinical environment. It has proven to be the best and fairest way to assess a student's competency to carry out the job of a doctor and will likely be used extensively to assess you at every stage of your medical career. It is best to familiarise yourself with the structure of the OSCE you will sit at your medical school. The OSCE tests a wide range of skills, with various different stations. This book will focus solely on the Medical History-Taking stations, which play a big part of the clinical curriculum and which you will undoubtedly be tested on, repeatedly.

Remember, you are being assessed by people, not robots. It is easy to fall into the trap of memorising lists of questions and series of steps from a textbook but the people assessing you will want to see a competent, caring individual who is not only knowledgeable but able to apply this knowledge in clinical practice, with the end goal of providing safe, compassionate patient care.

The History-taking station

The History-taking station of an OSCE aims to examine your communication skills and ability to take a 'medical history'. This is a conversation with the patient where you build a relationship and explore their current health problem, gathering as much information as possible to form a differential diagnosis, guide examinations and investigations, while seeking to rule out serious conditions which require urgent escalation.

You should actively listen to your patient and explore their physical and psychological health and wellbeing, including:
- Past or current medical conditions (incl. allergies) and treatments (incl. drug history);
- The physical and psychological health and wellbeing of the family;
- The patient's environment, social network and support;
- Any other factors influencing their health, provision of treatment and prevention of disease.

Usually, OSCE History-taking stations are structured to last 8 minutes in total, with a warning at 6 minutes. At this point, you may be asked to present the history you have just taken or simply your differential diagnosis and next steps. Structure your differential diagnosis from most to least likely and justify this with information from the history. Then suggest what you would consider doing for the patient, generally following the structure of Examinations and Investigations (Bedside tests, Bloods, Imaging, Special tests etc.). Finally, once you have fed back to the examiner all that is required, you can return to the history-taking! A lot of students are unaware of this and sit there in silence for the rest of the time – make sure you use this time to maximise those marks!

How to use this book

The best way to gain the most from this book is to let it guide your independent learning. Everything in this book is 'core knowledge' i.e. the absolute basic information you must have by the time you're a doctor. However, the top students will need to supplement this with some extra reading in order to really shine in their written exams.

1. Read through the **three frameworks** twice and memorise them
2. Read the **Presenting Complaint section that you're interested in**
3. Understand the main differential, investigations and treatment options
4. Put your new found knowledge to test by practicing with a partner using the example histories given

General Tips

- Read the vignette and make sure that you stick to what is relevant.

- Keep to time.

- Be nice to the patient – global marks are available for this.

- Manner is very important – you do not have a machine marking you, they are humans and, as such, will want to see a genuine human interaction rather than an automaton reeling off questions and facts.

- Use any spare time even after the 6-minute warning!

- Do not get phased by patients seeming off or unfriendly, if you manage to remain focused and efficient in your History-taking whilst still being warm and empathetic, this could really set you apart from the other candidates

- Practice different scenarios and don't be inflexible, especially as you become more confident, make sure you practice going in without a presenting complaint, for example – I have had real OSCE examinations where the vignette read: "This patient has come in with a complaint. Take a focused History" – if you have practiced by using the 2-minute vignette time to think of what you're about to ask, this could really throw you – be prepared!

- Make sure you prepare for different patients who may prefer different styles, something that is definitely not as black or white as medical schools make it seem. My university is quite keen on teaching students to start their history-taking with open questions to give the patient a chance to talk about whatever is troubling them, put them at ease, and combat the paternalistic approach to a medical interview that was common practice in the past. This is definitely the right way to approach your OSCE and clinical practice.

- However, I have had an OSCE examination which, after the standard introduction, went like this verbatim:
  - ➤ Me: Do you mind telling me what brings you in?
  - ➤ Patient: I've got some tummy pain.
  - ➤ Me: Can you tell me a little more about that?
  - ➤ Patient: What do you want to know?
  - ➤ Me: Whatever you'd like to tell me.
  - ➤ Patient: You're going to have to be more specific.

I really thought I needed to keep the history open at the start but this patient had different expectations. And so, I started asking specific, closed questions. The patient's feedback was that I shouldn't expect to be volunteered information but rather ask closed questions from the start to show that I know what I'm talking about rather than fishing for clues – the rest of the history went well once I started asking closed questions and I ended up having a high mark – which goes to show that if you remain focused you can overcome most things that could go wrong.

HISTORY FRAMEWORKS

The purpose of this chapter is to:

1) Introduce you to history-taking frameworks that you can **commit to memory** and use as a guide for most presenting complaints. This will make it significantly easier for you to come up with a sensible set of differential diagnosis and it will make your OSCE practice with others much more focused and efficient, so I highly recommend you memorise these before moving on to subsequent chapters.

2) Introduce you to a list of bodily systems, the ones you are likely to encounter at this stage, followed by a series of questions which aim to pick up on any problems the patient may have – if you pick up on anything, you can then ask subsequent questions. It is important to ask the questions even though they might not be related as, often, there are more marks available for ruling out alternative diagnoses than for simply getting to the right Dx based on intuition – leave that for the consultants!

The main frameworks to remember:
(1) The **GENERIC** framework (you can apply to most presenting complaints)

(2) The framework for **PAIN** (the "WOC SOCRATES" acronym is very useful to structure a history-taking when the patient comes in with pain *anywhere* in the body)

(3) The framework for most **CENTRAL NERVOUS SYSTEM** presenting complaints (for which it is useful to use the "WOC SOCRATES" acronym and several consultants recommend asking about Handedness – we can use "WOCH SOCRATES")

Top Tip:
As a rule, you can use a "WOC SOCRATES" based framework for most presenting complaints that refer to a specific <u>LOCATION</u> in the body E.g. Pain, Numbness, Headache, Lumps, etc

---

THE MAIN SYSTEMS TO COVER:

- Neurological
- Ophthalmological
- ENT
- Cardiovascular
- Respiratory
- Gastrointestinal

- Genitourinary
- Gynaecological
- Musculoskeletal
- Dermatological
- Constitutional

THE GENERAL FRAMEWORK

You can apply this framework to a number of presenting complaints and, if you're ever thrown by a presenting complaint you have never come across before, revert back to this! The framework alone should be enough for you to avoid awkward pauses and ask meaningful questions in a structured manner – and this should definitely allow for you to come up with a sensible differential diagnosis (and respective investigations).

"WIPE" – Introduce yourself, whilst gaining consent
o   Wash hands
o   Introduce self – "Hello, my name is X and I am a medical student"
o   Patient details – "Could I ask your full name and age?"
o   Explain – "I have been asked to speak with you about what brings you in, would that be alright?"

OPEN QUESTION (± CLARIFICATION) – to introduce yourself and put the patient at ease, helping to build rapport. The introduction will vary greatly from person to person but whatever you do, make sure it works for you (helping to set you apart as a strong candidate from the start) and ticks the boxes for available marks. I would recommend:
o   Hello, my name is X and I am a medical student. I have been asked to have a talk with you about what brings you in today, would that be okay?
o   If your vignette tells you what PC the patient has come in with, you could save yourself some time and be more direct with: "Hello, my name is X and I am a medical student. I understand you've come in with X, could you please tell me more about that?"

TIMELINE – Establishing a timeline will narrow down your differential diagnosis and well as hint at the severity of the presentation. Always ask these 5 questions:
1)   Start – When did this start? Did anything happen around then?
2)   Onset – Did it come on suddenly or gradually?
3)   Fluctuation – Does it come and go or is it there all the time?
4)   Progression – Has is changed at all? Has it gotten any better or worse?
5)   1st time – Have you had anything like this before?

SYMPTOMS – ask questions related to the presenting complaint –E.g.: Remember as: "MPS ROB"
1.   **Motion** – Do you find it difficult to initiate the swallow or swallowing itself?
2.   **Pain** – Do you have any pain when you swallow?
3.   **Smell** – Have you noticed bad breath recently?
4.   **Regurgitation** – Do you ever bring up food or drink after you've swallowed?
5.   **hOarseness** – Have you noticed any hoarseness in your voice?
6.   **Bulging/ Gargling** – any bulging of neck or gargling on eating?

SYSTEMS – review the systems of the body that could be related –
E.g.: Dysphagia
➢   **GI** – Appetite, Swallow, Vomiting, Tummy pain, Bowel motions, Stool changes
➢   **Neuro** – Headache, Change in any of the senses, Loss of sensation, Tingling/ pins & needles, Weakness?
➢   **(Anxiety** – Are you an anxious person? Do you think this could be related?)
➢   **Constitutional** – Appetite, Weight change, Tired, Fever, Night-sweats, Pains, rigidity

This completes the first part of the history, for which you should aim to spend about 65% of your time. You have now fully enquired about the presenting complaint and will hopefully have a pretty clear picture of what is going on. Now onto the second part, which is very similar for most presenting complaints, with a few nuances. Remember that there are marks for completing this second part but most of your information is likely to come from the first part. Don't, however, get too bogged down by this. Occasionally, you will find that by this point you've narrowed it down to a few possible diagnoses and this second part of the history may provide valuable information, especially in OSCEs where presentations are very stereotypical.

For example:

A patient who has come in with a relatively sudden onset headache. If they've come in with symptoms of meningism, by this point you *may* have narrowed it down to meningitis or a subarachnoid haemorrhage (SAH). If then, in the family history, it is mentioned they have a relative who passed away of a SAH or a relative affected by polycystic kidney disease (PCKD), then a SAH becomes the most likely diagnosis and you should mention this when presenting back to the examiner: "My top differential diagnosis is a SAH, due to the family history of polycystic kidney disease and the death of a first degree relative from 'a bleed in the brain'. However, due to the presentation of meningism, I would also like to rule out meningitis and other possible causes, such as...."

ICE – Elicit the patient's **I**deas, **C**oncerns, **E**xpectations, making sure they feel involved in the consultation (and consequently bringing up your patient marks) & allowing them to volunteer any information you may have missed.

➢ **Ideas** – You've given me a lot of information to work with, thank you for that. I'd like to know whether you have any idea what this could be.
➢ **Concerns** – Is anything concerning you that you would like to discuss?
➢ **Expectations** – What would you like to get from this consultation? (Resolution vs. Reassurance) (Not relevant for every PC, beware!)

PMHx
➢ Do you have any medical conditions?
➢ Ask specific questions pertaining to the diagnosis you have in mind – leaving it at a generic question risks missing valuable information if the patient chooses not to give information away

DHx
➢ Are you on any medication at the moment?
➢ Consider asking about over-the-counter or alternative/ herbal medicine
➢ Do you have any allergies?

FHx
➢ Are you aware of any conditions that run in the family?
➢ Has anyone in the family ever gone through anything similar to what you're going though?
➢ Ask specific questions if applicable

SHx – this can give you clues to the diagnosis and allows you to assess the support network available to your patient and make extra arrangements if needed
Remember it as 'SHO':
➢ **S**moking/ Alcohol/ Recreational drugs
➢ **H**ome environment? Support?
➢ **O**ccupation – impact of the condition on life and on occupation?

SUMMARISE & THANK – very important to wrap up the consultation nicely and transition smoothly into the presentation of the history to the examiner:
➢ Summarise if you have the time
➢ Is there anything you'd like to talk about that we haven't quite addressed?
➢ Thank you very much for talking to me and I wish you all the best

> **Summary:**
> - WIPE → Open ± Clarification
> - Timeline (x5) → Symptoms → Systems
> - ICE → PMHx →
> - DHx → FHx
> - SHx → Summarise & Thanks

THE PAIN FRAMEWORK
"WOCC SOCRATES"

"WIPE" – Introduce yourself, whilst gaining consent

a.   Wash hands

b.   Introduce self – "Hello, my name is X and I am a medical student"

c.   Patient details – "Could I ask your full name and age?"

d.   Explain – "I have been asked to speak with you about what brings you in, would that be alright?"

Open – Start with an open question:

a.   I understand you've come in with pain, do you mind telling me about that?

Clarification/ **C**onsider pain relief

a.   if anything is unclear: what exactly do you mean by…?

b.   If the actor seems to be in a lot of pain, briefly ask if they've been offered pain relief. This should put them at ease and help build rapport.

Site – Where exactly is the pain?

Onset – **Here you can use the same timeline you use in your general framework:**

A.   START – When did this start? Did anything happen around then?

B.   ONSET – Did it come on suddenly or gradually?

C.   FLUCTUATION – Does it come and go or is it there all the time?

D.   PROGRESSION – Has it changed? Has it gotten any better or worse?

E.   1st TIME – Have you ever had anything like this?

Character – Can you describe the pain for me? What does it feel like? (Sharp, dull, crushing, tearing, burning, etc.)

Radiation - Do you have this pain anywhere else?

Associated symptoms – **Here you can incorporate both SYMPTOMS and SYSTEMS:**

A.   Symptoms

   a.   Have you noticed any other changes in your body besides the pain?

   b.   Clarify anything about the pain and associated symptoms.

B.   Systems

   a.   Ask about body systems depending on the location of the pain.

   b.   E.g. Abdominal/ Tummy pain

1.   Cardiorespiratory – Chest pain, Breathlessness, Palpitations, cough

2.   Gastrointestinal – Appetite, Swallow, Vomiting, Tummy pain, Bowel habits, Stool changes

3.   Genitourinary – Waterworks, Pain, Colour, Frequency, Leakage, Urgency, LUTS

4.   Gynaecological – Sexually active, Pregnant, Last menstrual period

5.   Constitutional – Appetite, Weight change, Tired, Fever, Night-sweats, Pains or rigidity

Exacerbation/ Relief? – Have you noticed if anything makes the pain better or worse? (If you get a reply along the lines of "like what?", make sure to be specific – medications/ changes in position/ sleeping/ etc.)

Severity – How would you rate the pain on a scale of 1-10? 1 being not too bad and 10 being the worst pain imaginable.

ICE
a. Do you have any idea what could be causing the pain?
b. Is anything concerning you that you'd particularly like to discuss?
c. Is the main thing you seek from this consultation the resolution of the pain? Or reassurance?

PMHx
a. Do you have any medical conditions?
b. Ask specific questions pertaining to the diagnosis you have in mind – leaving it at a generic question risks missing valuable information if the patient chooses not to give information away

DHx
a. Are you on any medication at the moment?
b. Consider asking about over-the-counter or alternative/ herbal medicine
c. Some conditions could be triggered by medication
d. Do you have any allergies?

FHx
a. Are you aware of any conditions that run in the family?
b. Has anyone in the family ever gone through anything similar to what you're going though?
c. Ask specific questions if applicable

SHx – "SHO"
a. **S**moking/ Alcohol/ Recreational drugs
b. **H**ome environment? Support?
c. **O**ccupation – impact of the pain on life and on occupation?

SUMMARISE & THANK – very important to wrap up the consultation nicely and transition smoothly into the presentation of the history to the examiner:
a. Summarise if you have the time
b. Is there anything you'd like to talk about that we haven't quite addressed?
c. Thank you very much for talking to me and I wish you all the best

---

Summary:
- WIPE → Open ± Clarification
- Site & Onset → Character, Radiation & Associated Symptoms
- ICE
- PMHx → DHx
- FHx → SHx
- Summarise & Thanks

THE CNS FRAMEWORK
"WOCH SOCRATES"

"WIPE" – Introduce yourself, whilst gaining consent
> Wash hands
> Introduce self – "Hello, my name is X and I am a medical student"
> Patient details – "Could I ask your full name and age?"
> Explain – "I have been asked to speak with you about what brings you in, would that be alright?"

Open – Start with an open question:
> I understand you've come in with X, do you mind telling me about that?

Clarify – if anything is unclear: "What exactly do you mean by XYZ?"

Handedness – Before we go on, I'd like to ask whether you're right or left handed?

Site – Where exactly is the weakness?

Onset – **Here you can use the same timeline you use in your general framework:**
START – When did this start? Did anything happen around then?
ONSET – Did it come on suddenly or gradually?
FLUCTUATION – Does it come and go or is it there all the time?
PROGRESSION – Has it changed at all? Has it gotten any better or worse?
1st TIME – Have you ever had anything like this before?

Character – Can you describe the pain for me? What does it feel like? (Sharp, dull, crushing, tearing, burning, etc.)

Radiation – Does the weakness affect any other parts of your body?

Associated symptoms – **Here you can incorporate both SYMPTOMS and SYSTEMS:**
Symptoms
> Have you noticed any other changes in your body besides the pain?
> **Clarify anything about the pain and associated symptoms.**
Systems
Ask about body systems depending on the location of the pain.
E.g. Abdominal/ Tummy pain
> Cardiorespiratory – Chest pain, Breathlessness, Palpitations, cough
> Gastrointestinal – Appetite, Swallow, Vomiting, Tummy pain, Bowel habits, Stool changes
> Genitourinary – Waterworks, Pain, Colour, Frequency, Leakage, Urgency, LUTS
> Gynaecological – Sexually active, Pregnant, Last menstrual period
> Constitutional – Appetite, Weight change, Tired, Fever, Night-sweats, Pains or rigidity

Timing – This has been done.

Exacerbations/ Relief? – Have you noticed if anything makes the X better or worse? (If you get a reply along the lines of "like what?", make sure to be specific – medications/ changes in position/ sleeping/ etc.)

Severity – How badly is this affecting you?

ICE –
Do you have any idea what could be causing the pain?
Is anything concerning you that you'd particularly like to discuss?
Is the main thing you seek from this consultation the resolution of the pain? Or reassurance?

PMHx

Do you have any medical conditions?

Ask specific questions pertaining to the DDx you have in mind – leaving it at a generic question risks missing valuable information if the patient chooses not to give information away

DHx

Are you on any medication at the moment?

Consider asking about over-the-counter or alternative/ herbal medicine

Some conditions could be triggered by medication

Do you have any allergies?

FHx

Are you aware of any conditions that run in the family?

Has anyone in the family ever gone through anything similar to what you're going though?

Ask specific questions if applicable

SHx

Smoking/ Alcohol/ Recreational drugs

Home environment? Support?

Occupation – impact on life and on occupation?

SUMMARISE and THANK – it's important to wrap up the consultation and transition smoothly into the presentation of the history to the examiner

Summarise if you have the time

Is there anything you'd like to talk about that we haven't quite addressed?

Thank you very much for talking to me and I wish you all the best

THE SYSTEMS REVIEW

These following list of systems is structured as head to toe and then generalised, to make it easier to memorise. For each of them, I recommend that you memorise the following questions, which should be comprehensive enough to elicit most symptoms from the patient.

Neurological (remember as headache; senses; weakness)
1) Have you had a **headache**?
2) Have you noticed a change in **vision**? **Smell**? **Taste**?
3) Have you noticed a loss of **sensation**? Any **tingling/ pins & needles**?
4) Have you noticed any **weakness**?

Ophthalmological (remember as vision; sensation; appearance)
1) Have you noticed a change in **vision**?
2) Have you had any eye **pain**? **Itching**?
3) Have you noticed any **redness**? **Discharge**?

Ear, Nose, Throat
➤ Ear – 1) Any **ear pain**? 2) **Hearing loss**? 3) Any **Ringing**? 4) Any **discharge**?
➤ Nose – 5) Any **nose pain**? 6) **Bleed**? 7) **Discharge**?
➤ Throat – 8) **Pain**?

Cardiovascular (remember as pain; heart; breath; fluid)
1) Have you had any chest **pain**?
2) Have you noticed any **palpitations**? Awareness of your heartbeat?
3) Have you had any **loss of consciousness**? **Falls**?
4) Do you ever feel **breathless**?
5) Ever get **breathless at night**? How many **pillows** do you sleep with?
6) Have you noticed any **swelling** in your ankles or lower back?

Respiratory (remember as pain; breath; cough; wheeze)
1) Have you had any chest **pain**?
2) Do you ever feel **breathless**?
3) Have you had a **cough**? ± Any **blood**? ± Any **sputum**?
4) Have you heard any **wheezing** when you breathe?

Gastrointestinal (remember as head to toe)
1) How has your **appetite** been?
2) Have you had any problems **swallowing**?
3) Have you been **sick** at all? ±**blood**?
4) Have you had any tummy **pain**?
5) Have you noticed any change in your **bowel habits**?
6) A personal question. Have you noticed any changes in your **stool**?

Genitourinary
1) How have the **waterworks** been?
2) Have you had any **pain** on passing urine?
3) Have you noticed any changes in the **colour** of the urine?
4) Have you been passing urine more **frequently**? Increased **amounts**?
5) Do you ever **leak** urine? Feel an **urgent** need to pass urine?
6) Lower urinary tract symptoms:
    a) Do you have any difficulty passing urine?
    b) When you start passing urine, is it a continuous flow?
    c) Do you ever have any dribbling after passing urine?

Gynaecological – Remember to introduce as: "a few personal questions"
1) Are you **sexually active**?
2) Is there any chance you could be **pregnant**?
3) When was your **last menstrual period**?

Musculoskeletal –
1) Have you had any back or joint pain?
2) Have you experienced any stiffness?

Dermatological –
1) Any skin changes?
2) Rashes?
3) Ulcers?

Psychiatric –
1) How has your mood been?
2) Have you been feeling particularly anxious recently?

Constitutional –
1) How has your **appetite** been? Have you noticed a change in **weight**?
2) Have you been feeling especially **tired** recently?
3) Have you had a **fever**? Any **night-sweats**?
4) Have you had any **pains** or **rigidity** anywhere in your body?

Sexual –
1) A more personal question. Are you sexually active? 1 partner or multiple?
2) Any unprotected sexual intercourse?

Travel –
1) Have you travelled anywhere recently?

Histories Based On Presenting Complaint

This chapter includes a list of common presenting complaints, known to often come up in OSCEs at various medical schools – as well as a list of recommended questions which you could aim to remember – although you would probably be better off familiarising yourself with them at first and you will see that they often become quite intuitive, especially once you have memorised the generic History-taking framework.

When it comes to exploring SYMPTOMS and the SYSTEMS – don't worry too much if you don't manage to cover all the symptoms listed in this section for a particular presenting complaint. Likewise, don't worry if you get to the end of your SYMPTOMS exploration and have no idea what is going on. You can use your brief, systematic SYSTEMS review to not only rule out several presenting complaints but also narrow down your differential diagnosis significantly.

CENTRAL NERVOUS SYSTEM HISTORIES

HEADACHE
"WOC(C)H SOCRATES"

"**W**IPE" – Introduce yourself, whilst gaining consent
- Wash hands
- Introduce self – "Hello, my name is X and I am a medical student"
- Patient details – "Could I please ask your full name and age?"
- Explain – "I have been asked to speak with you about what brings you in, would that be alright?"

Open
- I understand you've come in with a headache could you tell me more about that?
- **C**larify
- **C**onsider pain relief – You seem to be in a lot of pain. Have you been offered pain relief?
- **H**andedness – "Before asking some more questions about this headache I'd just like to ask you whether you're left or right handed."

Site
- Where exactly is the headache? – site + uni or bilateral

Onset
1. When did it start? Did anything happen then?
2. Did it come on suddenly or gradually?
3. Does it come and go or is it always there?
4. Has it been getting worse?
5. Have you ever had a headache like this before?

Character
- Can you describe the pain? – pulsating, band around head, diffuse dull ache

Radiation
- Does the pain move anywhere?
    - ➢ Cluster = localised around 1 eye
    - ➢ Giant Cell Arteritis = temple/ jaw/ shoulder
    - ➢ Trigeminal neuralgia = face

Associated Symptoms
Symptoms – "MAT3R"
- Have you been ill or had a fever recently? (**M**eningitis)
- Did you have any warning that the headache was coming on? (**A**ura)
- Have you banged your head any time in the last few months? (**T**rauma) (Subdural –long lag/ Extradural – lucid interval)
- RULE OUT 3 **R**ED FLAGS!!
    - ➢ Any red eye? Haloes around bright lights? (AACG)
    - ➢ Any fever? Neck stiffness? Rashes? (Meningococcal septicaemia)
    - ➢ Any jaw pain on chewing? Scalp tenderness? (GCA)
Systems
- **Neurological** – Changes in sight? Hearing? Smell? Taste? Weakness? Altered sensation or pins & needles?
- **Musculoskeletal** – any joint or muscle pain or stiffness?
- **Constitutional** – Had any weight loss? Any fevers? Any night sweats?

Timing – This has been done.

Exacerbation/ Relief?
- Have you noticed if anything makes the pain better or worse?
- Is it worse when you cough/ strain/ lean forwards?
- Is it worse in dark or light?

Severity – How would you rate the pain on a scale of 1-10? 1 being not too bad and 10 being the worst pain imaginable.

ICE
- Do you have any idea what could be causing the pain?
- Is anything concerning you that you'd particularly like to discuss?
- Is the main thing you seek from this consultation the resolution of the pain? Or reassurance?

PMHx
- Do you have any medical conditions?
- Specifically, I'd like to ask if you've ever been diagnosed with:
  - ➢ Migraines? Polycystic kidney disease? A blood disorder? High BP? Any eye problems?

DHx
- Are you on any medication at the moment?
  - ➢ Any blood thinning medication?
- Consider asking about over-the-counter or alternative/ herbal medicine
- Do you have any allergies?

FHx
- Are you aware of any conditions that run in the family?
- Has anyone in the family ever gone through anything similar to what you're going though?
- Does anyone in the family have any kidney problems? Glaucoma? Migraines? Anyone ever had a bleed in the brain? Anyone had meningitis? Any FHx of sudden death?

SHx –
- Smoking/ Alcohol/ Recreational drugs
- Home environment? Support?
- Occupation – impact on life and on occupation?

Summarise and Thank
- I'd just like to summarise back to you to make sure I haven't missed anything
- Is there anything you'd like to talk about that we haven't quite addressed?
- Thank you for talking to me and I wish you all the best

Diagnosis	Features In History	Features In Investigations	Management
Migraine	Unilateral, throbbing, aura, may have a trigger, photo- and phono- phobia, helped by darkness and rest, nausea and vomiting	No findings	Trigger avoidance. Triptans may be useful if taken as soon as possible after onset
Meningitis	Prodromal illness, fever, neck stiffness, rash (non-blanching), photophobia	Kernig's positive on examination, non-blanching rash, raised WCC and CRP, positive blood and CSF cultures.	Admit to hospital. Immediate antibiotics
Cluster	Extreme pain, sudden onset, unilateral, periorbital, lacrimation, rhinorrhoea, same time daily for several days – weeks.	Nil	Abortive: oxygen, triptans Preventative: calcium channel blockers, mood stabilisers
Tension	Band around head, gradual onset, stress associated	Nil	NSAIDs
Sub-Arachnoid	Sudden onset, severe, occipital headache, meningism, reduced GCS, nausea, personal / family history of PKD	May see bleed on CT head if early. Xanthochromia in lumbar puncture or blood on CSF microscopy.	Neurosurgical management
Raised ICP	Morning headache, dull, worse on coughing and bending forwards, blurred vision, overweight	Papilloedema, large blind spot, CT head findings of raised pressure / tumour	Treat underlying cause
Giant Cell Arteritis	Unilateral, tender over temporal artery, worse with eating/combing hair, amaurosis fugax	Pulseless temporal artery, may feel lumps. Skip lesions in temporal artery biopsy	High dose steroids immediately if suspected and rheumatological follow up

Also Consider: Venous Sinus Thrombosis

Investigations

	General	Specific
Examination	Full neurological examination, including cranial nerves, ophthalmoscopy, Kernig's sign	
Bedside	Blood glucose, urine dip	
Bloods	FBC, U&E, CRP, ESR	Meningitis: blood cultures
Imaging	CT head	
Special	Lumbar puncture	GCA: temporal artery biopsy

	Site, Character & Radiation	Timing	Exacerbating and Relieving Factors	Associated Symptoms
Tension	"Band around head". Bilateral Non pulsing	Gradual onset Stress associated Stays the same	Stress Dehydration NSAIDs help	
Rebound	Bilateral non throbbing	After long term NSAID use	NSAIDs don't help	
Sinusitis	Over sinuses Dull, aching, tight	Gradual onset Constant Last weeks	Worse on bending over and movement, Sneezing, coughing	Coryzal symptoms Tender overlying skin Post nasal drip
Migraine	Unilateral Throbbing	Prodromal (days-hrs), aura (just before), headache, post-dromal Last 2-72hrs Recurrent	Triggers: cheese, OCP, caffeine, alcohol. Light and sounds worsen. Darkness and rest help.	Aura just before (not necessary): Visual / somatosensory symptoms Paraesthesia / motor Nausea and vomiting
Trigeminal Neuralgia	Unilateral stabbing in CN V distribution	Paroxysmal Sudden Lasts seconds	Stimulating the area (shaving, washing, touching, eating)	Tic doloreux (face screwed up in pain)
Cluster Headache	Unilateral Periorbital Severe	Sudden onset 15-180 mins Clusters of regular headaches for up to a month with remission up to years long		Conjunctival injection, lacrimation, nasal congestion, rhinorrhoea, facial sweating, miosis, ptosis, or eyelid oedema
Temporal Arteritis	Unilateral Tender over temporal art.	Sub-acute onset Weeks duration. Eating/combing hair can trigger	Chewing makes worse	Pulseless temporal artery Jaw claudication Amaurosis Fugax
Raised ICP	Dull Generalised	Persistent Worst in morning	Worse on coughing, Valsalva, bending over	Papilloedema Vomiting Seizures Focal neurological signs if tumour
Acute Glaucoma	Unilateral Aching Radiates to forehead	Constant Precipitated by sitting in dark (cinema)		Acutely reduced vision, Visual halo & red eye Cloudy cornea Dilated non responsive pupil
Subdural		May be sudden onset Usually insidious after initial trauma	Maybe worse: coughing, straining, exercise	Decreased consciousness Motor or cognitive losses N+V RF: falls, anticoagulants
Extra-Dural	Unilateral	Following trauma LOC, lucid interval then slow decline in consciousness → coma	As raised ICP	Cushing's triad (bradycardia, irregular breathing, hypertension) N+V
Encephalitis or Meningitis	Generalised Severe	Pro-dromal viral illness (VZV, EBV, CMV, measles, mumps) Hours - days	Photophobia	Fever Lethargy Seizures Neck Stiffness & Rash (Meningitis only) Confusion or personality changes (Encephalitis only)
Sub-Arachnoid	Severe – "worst ever" Occipital	Thunderclap		Focal Neurological Signs Decreased consciousness Nausea & Vomiting Associated with PKD

Marking Criteria HEADACHE	Marks	
	Awarded	Available
Washed hands at the start of the station		1
Introduced themselves – Including First name, last name and role		1
Patient details confirmed: Full name, Age/ D.O.B.		1
Explained purpose of consultation		1
Open question about what brings the patient in today + Clarification of any ambiguity		1
Site – Enquires about exact location of headache - Uni/ Bi, Localised/ Diffuse, etc.		1
Onset (Timeline) – Asks questions to provide a clear understanding of onset and progression - Onset/ Circumstance - Sudden vs. gradual - Fluctuations - Progression - Past episodes		3
Character - Obtains an accurate description of the headache		1
Radiation - Asks about the pain moving anywhere else		1
Associated symptoms ▪ **Symptoms** elicited are relevant and clearly directed at either arriving at a diagnosis or excluding other plausible diagnoses - Aura - Meningitis - Symptom lag time/ Lucid interval - MUST rule out 3 red flags – AACG, Meningococcal septicaemia, GCA **(If omitted award 0 marks for Symptoms section)** ▪ **Systems** queried are relevant to the complaint and adequate questions are asked for each symptom - Neurological; Musculoskeletal; Constitutional		6
Timing - This has been done		0
Exacerbation/ Relief - Clearly asks if the patient has noticed any relieving/ exacerbating factors, providing appropriate examples if prompted (Ex. Straining, posture, hot/ cold)		1
Severity - Subjective quantitative assessment of headache severity		1
Explores **Ideas, Concerns and Expectations**		3
Elicits relevant **Past Medical History** - Migraine; PCKD; Bleeding disorder; HTN; Eye problems		2
Elicits relevant **Drug History** including **Allergies**		2
Elicits relevant **Family History**		2
Elicits relevant **Social History** – including Smoking/ alcohol/ recreational drugs; Home environment and support; Occupation and impact on life		2
Closes consultation appropriately allowing the patient to ask any questions		1
Presentation: structured, concise		2
Appropriate Differential Diagnosis ± Investigations ± Management Plan		3
Examiner mark – professionalism and rapport		5
Patient mark – professionalism and rapport		5

Consultation	Presentation	Global marks patient	Global marks examiner	Total
30	5	5	5	45

35-year-old Female severe headache for 18 hours

HPC	Severe headache since yesterday afternoon Initially some visual disturbance followed by severe headache mainly on the left side, throbbing type, never had such severe pain, accompanied by nausea, followed by weakness to arm followed by leg. Not relieved with the pain killers or going to dark room. Going through lot of stress recently and not able to sleep in the night for last 5 days Used to have mild headache followed by visual disturbance, relived within hour after taking pain killer or going to dark room. Once or twice a year
PMH	Irritable bowel syndrome, anxiety
DH	Mebeverine
FH	Father had stroke 10 years ago, one of the uncle diagnosed as brain tumour recently
SH	Working as secretary, non-smoker and occasional alcohol, likes chocolate and cheese
ICE	Pain to get relived, do I have tumour/stroke
Dx	Hemiplegic Migraine on the basis of typical history (marching symptoms),
Ix	MRI head
Mx	Sumatriptan, analgesics prophylactic medication like b blocker, topiramate, pizotifen, prevention advice: decrease quantity of cheese, chocolate, flashing light and stress

55-year-old Male progressive headache for last one month

HPC	Frontal headache from one month, initially relieved with analgesics, now diffuse only responding slightly with analgesics, severe intensity, difficult to concentrate, causing intermittent confusion, wake of in the night due to severe intensity headache, sleepless night, now from last one week unsteady, dizzy with severe nausea, from last 2 days weakness of left side with speech problem, not able to work for last 3 weeks, not going through stress, no visual disturbance, still able to go out from home Has seen doctors before advised to take analgesics
PMH	Hypertension, hypothyroidism, intermittent palpitation never investigated
DH	Losartan, thyroxine, propranolol
FH	Mother had hypertension, Father had stroke at 75 years and died
SH	Working as builder, non-smoker, drink 6 pints over weekend
ICE	My head is exploding, is something wrong with me
Dx	Brain Tumour (rapidly progressing likely Glioblastoma),
Ix	CT Head/MRI Head (Contrast)
Mx	Analgesics, steroid, brain biopsy, Neurosurgery/MDT referral

40-year-old male

HPC	Severe headache for last 6 hours, initially frontal but now going to the neck, sudden onset, worst headache of life like thunderclap, developed while doing exercise in the gym, accompanied by nausea, dizziness with feeling of passing out, no limb weakness or fall with loss of vision or double vision, no loss of consciousness Taken paracetamol but no relieved
PMH	Polycystic kidney disease (not under any active follow up
DH	Hypertension (diet control), occasional paracetamol
FH	Father died of intracerebral bleed while he was 57 years old
SH	Works as banker, non-smoker, occasional alcohol
ICE	Headache is killing me and needs strong analgesics
Dx	Subarachnoid Haemorrhage
Ix	CT head/ may require lumbar puncture, CT head Circle of Willis angiogram
Mx	Neuro observation, coiling or clipping (bed rest, plenty of fluid and Nimodipine if on conservative pathway)

60-year-old male

HPC	Woke up in morning with severe pain on the back of head, feeing unsteady, nausea and difficulty to identify object on the left side, no weakness of the limbs, no speech or swallowing deficit, visited emergency department after 6 hours of feeling these symptoms, from 6 weeks having intermittent palpitation but no chest pain Never had like these symptoms before
PMH	Hypertension, Hypercholesterolemia
DH	Simvastatin 10 mg, Amlodipine
FH	Father had hypertension when he was 75 years old
SH	Working as accountant, smoker 10/day, occasional alcohol
ICE	Why my symptoms are getting better
Dx	Posterior circulation stroke secondary to atrial fibrillation
Ix	CT Head/MRI head, ECG, Bloods for cholesterol and glucose
Mx	Transfer to stroke unit, monitoring, aspirin, analgesics, multidisciplinary input, eye referral, later anticoagulatory drugs

75-year-old Male

HPC	Pain on the left side head for last one-week, constant headache but the severity varies, pain increases on pressing that area, also on hair combing, neck pain, low grade fever from last one week, neck pain and jaw claudication, transient vision loss of left eye, no weakness of limbs or swallowing or speech deficit, not responding to analgesics, recently to optician but no deficit except mild cataract, no morning stiffness
PMH	Hypertension, diabetes, cataract (but not operated)
DH	Gliclazide, Metformin, Amlodipine
FH	Both parents have died
SH	Retired, ex-smoker left 15 years back, occasional alcohol
ICE	Concern regarding transient sudden loss of vision am I going to become blind
Dx	Giant Cell Arteritis
Ix	Bloods like FBC, ESR, CRP, LFTs, CT head, temporal artery biopsy
Mx	Steroid, Rheumatology and eye clinic referral

40-year-old female

HPC	Several days of worsening headache. Sudden onset worsening and left sided facial droop. Patient complaining of left sided weakness. When presenting to hospital, she has difficulties speaking and articulating. Her voice sounds slurred. Patient also complains of visual disturbances and blurred vision.
PMH	Inflammatory bowel disease, sickle cell anaemia
DH	NKDA, oestrogen oral contraception, otherwise nil regular
FH	Adopted. Unknown family Hx
SH	Patient works in retail. Non-smoker. Social alcohol.
ICE	"My head feels like it's exploding and I can't see. I just want to be out of pain"
Dx	Cerebral Venous Sinus Thrombosis
Ix	CT head/MRI head, consider CT angiography, FBC, U&E, LFT, CRP, D-Dimer
Mx	Heparin, warfarin, consider thrombolysis, consider therapeutic LP if raised ICP, anticonvulsants to prevent seizures.

EYE PAIN
"WOCC SOCRATES"

"**W**IPE" – Introduce yourself, whilst gaining consent
- Wash hands
- Introduce self – "Hello, my name is X and I am a medical student"
- Patient details – "Could I ask your full name and age?"
- Explain – "I have been asked to speak with you about what brings you in, would that be alright?"

Open
- I understand you've come in with eye pain is that correct? Could you tell me more about that?
- **C**larify
- **C**onsider pain relief – You seem to be in a lot of pain. Have you been offered pain relief?

Site
- Where exactly is the pain? (Uni or bilateral)

Onset
1. When did the pain start? Did anything happen then?
2. Did it come on suddenly or gradually?
3. Does it come and go or is it always there?
4. Has it been getting worse over time?
5. Have you ever had anything like this before?

Character
- What does the pain feel like? Stabbing, diffuse dull ache?

Radiation
- Does this pain go anywhere else?

Associated symptoms
Symptoms – "DDIV3RRT"
- Have you noticed any **D**ryness?
- Have you had any **D**ischarge? **I**tching? (Conjunctivitis)
- Have you noticed a change in your **V**ision?
- RULE OUT 3 **R**ED FLAGS
  ➢ Any red eye? Haloes around bright lights? (AACG)
  ➢ Any jaw pain on chewing? Scalp tenderness? (GCA)
  ➢ Excruciating pain? Red eye? Photophobia? (Scleritis)
  ➢ Are you long or short sighted? (**R**efractive error) (hypermetropia = +AACG risk)
  ➢ Any **T**rauma to the eye? (Keratitis)

Systems
- **Respiratory** – Any SOB? Cough?
- **Gastrointestinal** – Any tummy pain? Change in your bowels? Stool?
- **Genitourinary** – How are the waterworks? Any pain on urination?
- **Musculoskeletal** – Any joint or back pain or stiffness?
- **Constitutional** – Had any weight loss? Any fevers? Any night sweats?

<u>T</u>iming – This has been done.

<u>E</u>xacerbation/ Relief?
- Have you noticed if anything makes the pain better or worse?
- Is it worse with dark? Bright lights? Contact with pets?
- Is it relieved by a cold compress?

<u>S</u>everity – How would you rate the pain on a scale of 1-10? 1 being not too bad and 10 being the worst pain imaginable.

ICE
- Do you have any idea what could be causing the pain?
- Is anything concerning you that you'd particularly like to discuss?
- Is the main thing you seek from this consultation the resolution of the pain? Or reassurance?

PMHx
- Do you have any medical conditions?
- Specifically, I'd like to ask if you've ever been diagnosed with:
  - ➢ Migraines? Something called an autoimmune condition? Arthritis? Any bowel conditions? Any STIs? High BP? Any eye problems?

DHx
- Are you on any medication at the moment?
- Consider asking about over-the-counter or alternative/ herbal medicine
- Do you have any allergies?

FHx
- Are you aware of any conditions that run in the family?
- Has anyone in the family ever gone through anything similar to what you're going though?
- Does anyone in the family have any eye problems? Specifically, glaucoma? Dry eye?

SHx –
- Smoking/ Alcohol/ Recreational drugs
- Home environment? Support?
- Occupation – impact on life and on occupation?

Summarise and Thank
- I'd just like to summarise back to you to make sure I haven't missed anything
- Is there anything you'd like to talk about that we haven't quite addressed?
- Thank you for talking to me and I wish you all the best

Differential Diagnosis

Diagnosis	Features In History	Features In Investigations	Management
Glaucoma	Pain (especially after being in darkness), severe, unilateral, blurred vision, N&V	Increased intraocular pressure, red eye, fixed pupil	Admit for ophthalmology assessment Pilocarpine eye drops, acetazolomide
Conjunctivitis	Itchy, irritated eye, foreign body sensation, watery, discharge, contact lens wearer	Red eye, lacrimation, conjunctival injection, normal acuity	Chloramphenicol eye drops, eye care advice, avoid contact lenses
Inflammatory	Systemic upset: fevers, arthralgia, history of IBD, skin rashes, history of STIs, Trauma or foreign body	Red eye, rash, arthralgia, arthritis. Raised CRP, ESR.	Treat underlying cause – antibiotics / anti-inflammatories

Investigations

	General	Specific
Bedside	Cranial nerve exam, fundoscopy	Thyroid: proptosis, exophthalmos, gaze palsy Systemic inflammatory: joint and skin examination, lymphadenopathy, rash
Bloods	FBC, U&E, CRP	Thyroid: TFTs Systemic: Connective tissue/Auto-antibody screen
Imaging	Consider CT head / MRI head and orbits	
Special	Slit lamp examination, intra ocular pressure	

Marking Criteria EYE PAIN	Marks	
	Awarded	Available
Washed hands at the start of the station		1
Introduced themselves – Including First name, last name and role		1
Patient details confirmed: Full name, Age/ D.O.B.		1
Explained purpose of consultation		1
Open question about what brings the patient in today + Clarification of any ambiguity		1
Site – Enquired about exact location of eye pain - Uni/ Bi, Localised/ Diffuse, etc.		1
Onset (Timeline) – Asked questions to provide a clear understanding of onset and progression - Onset/ Circumstance - Sudden vs. gradual - Fluctuations - Progression - Past episodes		3
Character - Obtained an accurate description of the eye pain		1
Radiation - Ask about the pain moving anywhere else – Ex. Temple, other eye, etc.		1
Associated symptoms ▪ **Symptoms** elicited are relevant and clearly directed at either arriving at a diagnosis or excluding other plausible diagnoses - **"DDIV3RRT"** o Dry; Discharge; Itch; Vision; 3R (AACG, GCA, Scleritis); Refract; Trauma **(If 3 red flags omitted award 0 marks for Symptoms section)** ▪ **Systems** queried are relevant to the complaint and adequate questions are asked for each symptom - Respiratory; Gastrointestinal; Genitourinary; Musculoskeletal; Constitutional		6
Timing - This has been done		0
Exacerbation/ Relief - Clearly asks if the patient has noticed any relieving/ exacerbating factors, providing appropriate examples if prompted (Ex. Lighting, pets, hot/ cold)		1
Severity - Subjective quantitative assessment of pain severity		1
Explores **Ideas, Concerns and Expectations**		3
Elicits relevant **Past Medical History** - Migraine; Autoimmune disorders; Arthritis; Bowel conditions; Sensitively enquire about STIs; HTN; Eye problems generally		2
Elicits relevant **Drug History** including **Allergies**		2
Elicits relevant **Family History**		2
Elicits relevant **Social History** – including Smoking/ alcohol/ recreational drugs; **H**ome environment and support; **O**ccupation and impact on life		2
Closes consultation appropriately allowing the patient to ask any questions		1
Presentation: structured, concise		2
Appropriate Differential Diagnosis ± Investigations ± Management Plan		3
Examiner mark – professionalism and rapport		5
Patient mark – professionalism and rapport		5

Consultation	Presentation	Global marks patient	Global marks examiner	Total
30	5	5	5	45

35-year-old male

HPC	Developed redness of eyes with pain and continuous irritation for one day, no history of any foreign body or using contact lens, burning urine with increased frequency of urine for last 6 days, recent diarrhoea, right knee pain and back pain for last 4 days, no skin lesion, no history of urethral discharge, no fever, no sexual history other than with partner
PMH	Had meningitis 2 years ago
DH	Taking paracetamol and chloramphenicol eye drops
FH	Father has Rheumatoid Arthritis when he was 35 years old
SH	Works as teacher, non-smoker, steady partner, occasional alcohol
ICE	Why all three things has come together
Dx	Reiter syndrome
Ix	ESR, urine culture, check for HLA B27
Mx	NSAID, steroid eye drop, steroid or disease modifying drug if symptoms not responding, symptoms may last for 2 weeks to 6 months. May have recurrent episode of arthritis

25-year-old female

HPC	Eyes pain involving both eyes from last 3 to 4 days, now light hurting as well as yellowish discharge, eyes has become red with local swelling, having cough cold for last one week, not using any contact lens with no history of allergies, has one steady partner, no history of trauma Symptoms worsen from last 3 to 4 days
PMH	Not significant
DH	Oral contraceptive, started oral antibiotics one day before for upper respiratory infection
FH	Not significant
SH	Work as a teacher assistant, smokes 5 cigarettes per day, does not take alcohol, has one steady partner
ICE	What is happening to my eyes?
Dx	Conjunctivitis (Bacterial)
Ix	Conjunctival scrapings and cultures (if severe)
Mx	Topical antibiotics

70-year-old female

HPC	Sudden onset of left eye pain with reddening for last a few hours, blurring of the vision headache mainly on left side, feels nauseous, had mild cataract with regular optician check, no history of foreign body Never had such pain in the eye and has taken Paracetamol but no relief
PMH	Mild cataract, hypertension
DH	Lisinopril, amlodipine
FH	My one of the brother developed similar condition when he was 70 years old
SH	Retired, non-smoker, no alcohol, enjoys doing gardening
ICE	This pain is killing me
Dx	Acute primary angle-closure glaucoma
Ix	Tonometry to check pressure, slit lamp examination ophthalmoscopy
Mx	Keep patient supine, Acetazolamide, B blocker eye drop like timolol, steroid eye drop, analgesics, antiemetic, Pilocarpine, laser peripheral iridotomy once pressure is controlled in 1 to 2 days

CHANGES IN VISION
GENERAL FRAMEWORK

<u>**"WIPE"**</u> – Introduce yourself, whilst gaining consent
- Wash hands
- Introduce self – "Hello, my name is X and I am a medical student"
- Patient details – "Could I ask your full name and age?"
- Explain – "I have been asked to speak with you about what brings you in, would that be alright?"

<u>**Open**</u>
- I understand you've come in with some problems seeing, do you mind telling me about that?
- Clarify – Do you know it this affects one eye or both? Have you tried covering it?
- **H**andedness – "Before asking some more questions about these vision problems, I'd just like to ask you whether you're left or right handed."

<u>**Timeline**</u>
1. When did this start?
2. Did it come on suddenly or gradually?
3. Does the loss of vision come and go or is it there all the time?
4. Has your vision been getting worse? Gradually?
5. Have you ever had vision problems like this before?

<u>**Symptoms**</u>
Sight loss
- You've already established whether one eye or both
- Where exactly is the sight loss? If I were to divide your vision into four **quadrants**, where exactly is sight impaired?
- What about the **centre versus outside**, which is affected more?
- **How bad** is this loss of vision? Can you see in this/ these corners at all?

Eyes – "PG DDIFF3RRT"
- **P**ain – Have you experienced any pain in your eyes?
- **G**lare – Do you notice a glare around bright lights?
- **D**ouble vision – Have you experienced any double vision?
- **D**ischarge – Any discharge from your eye?
- **I**tch – Any itching in your eye?
- **F**loaters – Have you noticed any objects floating in your field of vision?
- **F**lashes – Have you noticed any flashing of bright lights?
- RULE OUT **3 R**ED FLAGS
  - ➤ Any red eye? Haloes around bright lights? (AACG)
  - ➤ Any Excruciating pain? Red eye? Photophobia (Scleritis)
  - ➤ jaw pain on chewing? Scalp tenderness? (GCA)
- **R**efraction – Are you long or short sighted?
- **T**rauma – Is there any chance you might have injured your eyes?

<u>**Systems**</u>
- **Neurological** – Any headaches? Change smell, taste, hearing? Weakness? Weird sensation anywhere in your body?
- **Cardiovascular**– Have you had any chest pain/ discomfort? Any palpitations? Any LOC? Any SOB?

ICE
- You've given me a lot of information, thank you. I'd like to hear a little about what you think could be going on. Do you have any idea?
- Is there anything that's particularly concerning you that you'd like to discuss?
- What exactly are you looking for today, resolution or reassurance?

PMHx
- Do you have any medical conditions?
- Ask a few specific questions to show that you're thinking about different causes
- Specifically, I'd like to ask if you've ever been diagnosed with:
    - ➢ (CV risk factors) Diabetes? High blood pressure? Heart problems? Ever had a stroke or transient ischaemic attack?

DHx
- On any medication? Any doses of medication changed?
- Any allergies?

FHx
- Any conditions run in the family? Specifically, Diabetes; Glaucoma
- Has anyone in the family ever had problems with their vision?

SHx –
- Smoking/ Alcohol/ Recreational drugs
- Home environment? Support?
- Occupation – impact on life and on occupation?

Summarise and Thank
- I'd just like to summarise back to you to make sure I haven't missed anything
- Is there anything you'd like to talk about that we haven't quite addressed?
- Thank you for talking to me and I wish you all the best

Investigations

Examination	Cranial nerve exam, fundoscopy
Bedside	Blood glucose, blood pressure
Bloods	FBC, U&E, CRP, ESR, HbA1c, lipid profile, TFTs
Imaging	CT head +/- MRI head and orbits
Special	Slit lamp examination, intra-ocular pressures, carotid artery ultrasound Doppler, CSF analysis, temporal artery biopsy

Diagnosis	Features In History	Features In Investigations	Management
OCULAR	Corneal Scarring Recurrent corneal scarring/infections, contact lenses, herpetic ulcers, gradual loss, discharge	High uptake on fluorescein staining, dendritic herpetic ulcers with slit lamp	Ophthalmological management Glaucoma: pilocarpine
	Glaucoma Eye pain, history of haloes around lights	Raised intraocular pressure	
	Vitreous Haemorrhage Trauma, floaters, sudden, poor diabetes control	Loss of red reflex, decreased acuity, unable to visualise fundus, raised HbA1c	
	Retinal Detachment Trauma, curtain falling, flashes, floaters, distorted vision	Loss of red reflex, torn/crumpled retina on fundoscopy	
NEUROLOGICAL	Optic Neuritis Painful, unilateral, photophobia, temporary vision loss/ change in colour vision, other episodes of neuro symptoms (history of MS)	Oligoclonal bands on CSF in MS, demyelination on MRI head and spinal cord	Neurological / neurosurgical referral Consider steroids to reduce inflammation in acute setting (MS and tumours)
	Optic chiasm Loss of peripheral vision, raised ICP symptoms, pituitary tumour symptoms	Reduced visual fields peripherally, mass on CT head, raised pituitary hormones (prolactin)	
	Tumours Compression on optic tract – hemi/quadrantanopia	Cranial nerve VI palsy, mass on CT head	
VASCULAR	Retinal artery occlusion Sudden onset, painless, persistent, whole visual field, history of: IHD, diabetes, high cholesterol, AF, coagulopathy	Raised blood pressure, high HbA1c, high lipids, coagulopathy	Urgent referral to nearest stroke centre
	Retinal vein occlusion Redness, painful, watery, hypertension, diabetes		

Marking Criteria VISUAL CHANGES	Marks	
	Awarded	Available
Washed hands at the start of the station		1
Introduced themselves – Including First name, last name and role		1
Patient details confirmed: Full name, Age/ D.O.B.		1
Explained purpose of consultation		1
Open question about what brings the patient in today + Clarification of any ambiguity – E.g. Does this affect 1 eye or both? Have you checked by covering your eye?		1

Timeline allows a clear understanding of onset and progression of visual changes
  - Onset/ Circumstance
  - Sudden vs. gradual
  - Fluctuations
  - Progression
  - Past episodes
		3

Symptoms elicited are relevant and clearly directed at either arriving at a diagnosis or excluding other plausible diagnoses
  - Sight loss
    o Visual field affected – Ex. Quadrants; Central vs. peripheral vision
  - Eyes
    o Pain; Trauma; Glasses; Floaters; Flashes; Glare; Double vision
    o Rule out red flags! AACG; GCA
    (If omitted award 0 marks for Symptoms section)
		5

Systems queried are relevant to the complaint and adequate questions are asked for each symptom - Neurological; Cardiovascular		5
Explores **Ideas, Concerns and Expectations**		3
Elicits relevant **Past Medical History** - DM; HTN; Heart problems (esp. AF); Previous stroke or TIA		2
Elicits relevant **Drug History** including **Allergies**		2
Elicits relevant **Family History**		2
Elicits relevant **Social History** – including Smoking/ alcohol/ recreational drugs; **Home** environment and support; **Occupation** and impact on life		2
Closes consultation appropriately allowing the patient to ask any questions		1
Presentation: structured, concise		2
Appropriate Differential Diagnosis ± Investigations ± Management Plan		3
Examiner mark – professionalism and rapport		5
Patient mark – professionalism and rapport		5

Consultation	Presentation	Global marks patient	Global marks examiner	Total
30	5	5	5	45

72-year-old male

HPC	Sudden loss of vision involving the left eye, cannot see at all with this eye, no history of injury, intermittent palpitation, no chest pain, last optician check 2 months back, no obvious abnormality, taking regular medications as advised by doctor
PMH	Diabetes, Hypertension, Ischemic Heart disease, Hypercholesterolemia
DH	Aspirin, gliclazide, bisoprolol, ramipril, GTN spray, Atorvastatin
FH	Brother has early cataract and hypertension
SH	Retired, does some charity work, ex-smoker left 15 years back, no alcohol
ICE	Will my vision come back
Dx	Retinal artery occlusion
Ix	Eye clinic opinion, ECG, CT head, Carotid Doppler, check blood for glucose, TFT and cholesterol, 24-hour tape
Mx	Address the secondary risk factor for stroke, Clopidogrel, reassurance, monitor for depression

17-year-old male with rapid onset blurred vision

HPC	Rapid onset blurred vision in left eye. Patient says he can see flashes of light and feels like he is seeing more floaters than usually. Finds it difficult to walk down busy roads as he tends to not see people walking close to his side. Feels like there is a curtain over part of his visual field. Reports having been in a bar fight 3 weeks ago and being punched on the left side of his face.
PMH	Nil
DH	Nil regular. Occasional paracetamol and ibuprofen. NKDA
FH	Mother has T1DM, father is overweight.
SH	Student. 20 pack year smoker. Exercises regularly. Drinks 35 units per week, mostly on weekends with his mates
ICE	"I can't see properly when I'm at school, doctor"
Dx	Retinal detachment.
Ix	Ophthalmology appointment, slit lamp examination, examination for lymph nodes, FBC, U&E, CRP, fluorescein stain of cornea, measure intra-ocular pressure, ophthalmoscopy
Mx	Cryopexy and laser photocoagulation, scleral buckle surgery, pneumatic retinopexy, vitrectomy. Advise patient that injury can lead to permanent loss of vision if left untreated.

25-year-old male with visual light sensitivity

HPC	Patient reports sudden onset of pain and light sensitivity of the eye. He reports that he feels as if he has a foreign object in his eyes. Reports having washed his eyes out, but no improvement. Increased tear production. Reports no trauma or injury.
PMH	Appendectomy age 9, nil other
DH	NKDA, nil regular, occasional pain relief
FH	Nil.
SH	Works in construction as metalworker, drinks socially, smokes 10 per day.
ICE	"I need to get back to work, doctor and I can't do my job if I can't see properly."
Dx	Corneal Abrasion
Ix	Ophthalmoscopy, slit lamp microscopy, fluorescein shows scratches under cobalt blue-light
Mx	Topical tetracaine for pain, consider antibiotics if fear of contamination with bacterial matter.

PUPIL AND EYE CHANGES
GENERAL FRAMEWORK

"WIPE" – Introduce yourself, whilst gaining consent
- Wash hands
- Introduce self – "Hello, my name is X and I am a medical student"
- Patient details – "Could I ask your full name and age?"
- Explain – I have been asked to speak with you about what brings you in, would that be alright?

Open
- I understand you've come in because you're worried about your eye(s), do you mind telling me more about that?
- Clarify –

Timeline
1. When did you first notice this change in your eye?
2. Did it come on suddenly or gradually?
3. Does this come and go or is it there all the time?
4. Has is been getting worse?
5. Have you ever experienced anything like this before?

Symptoms
- **"P DIVRRT"**
- **P**ain – Have you had any pain in your eyes?
- **D**ischarge – Have you had any discharge from your eyes?
- **I**tching – Have you noticed any itching in your eyes?
- **V**ision – Have you had any problems seeing?
- **R**edness – Have you noticed any redness in your eyes? Whole eye? Part?
- **R**efraction – Are you long or short sighted?
- **T**rauma – Is there any chance you could have injured your eyes?

Systems
- **Neurological** – Have you had a headache? Noticed a change in any of your senses? And what about any weakness or altered sensation?
- **Constitutional** – Have you felt tired? Loss of appetite? Weight loss?

ICE
- You've given me a lot of information, thank you. I'd like to hear a little about what you think could be going on. Do you have any idea?
- Is there anything that's particularly concerning you that you'd like to discuss?
- What exactly are you looking for today, resolution or reassurance?

PMHx
- Do you have any medical conditions?
- Ask a few specific questions to show that you're thinking about different causes
- Specifically, I'd like to ask if you've ever been diagnosed with:
    - Diabetes? High blood pressure? Heart problems? Something called an autoimmune condition? Cancer?

DHx
- On any medication? Any doses of medication changed?
    - Specifically, are you on any blood thinning medication?
- Any allergies?

<u>**FHx**</u>
- Any conditions run in the family?
- Has anyone in the family ever had problems with their eyes?

<u>**SHx**</u> –
- Smoking/ Alcohol/ Recreational drugs
- Home environment? Support?
- Occupation – impact on life and on occupation?

<u>**Summarise and Thank**</u>
- I'd just like to summarise back to you to make sure I haven't missed anything
- Is there anything you'd like to talk about that we haven't quite addressed?
- Thank you for talking to me and I wish you all the be

<u>**Investigations**</u>

	General	**Specific**
Examination	Full cranial nerve examination, fundoscopy, chest examination	<u>Myasthenia gravis:</u> Repeated movements reduce in amplitude
Bedside		<u>Infection:</u> Swab discharge
Bloods	FBC, CRP, ESR, drug levels	
Imaging	CXR, CT head	
Special	Slit lamp exam	

Differential Diagnosis

Diagnosis	Features In History	Features In Investigations	Management
Ptosis	Myasthenia gravis Worse at end of day, associated dysphagia, soft voice	(Tensilon test), reduced amplitude of repeated movements	Anti-cholinesterases (pyridostygmine) Monitor respiratory function
	Horner's Unilateral, dry face, B-symptoms	Miosis, CXR for apical mass	Underlying cause if found – cancer therapy
	Bell's palsy Drooping of facial muscles, dry eye, ear herpetic lesions / infection, parotid enlargement	History of facial herpes (Ramsay-Hunt syndrome), compression along facial nerve pathway, parotid pathology	Anti-virals (Acyclovir) if within **72 hours** of onset with steroids or observe and treat underlying cause if found.
	Myopathies, CN III lesion/ compression	Weakness of muscle groups globally	
Redness	Conjunctivitis Redness, infection, foreign body, discharge	Discharge (swab shows bacteria)	Chloramphenicol eye drops / ointment
	Inflammatory Redness of conjunctiva, just around iris, ulcer on sclera, systemic upset, arthralgia, rashes, chronic breathing issues	Raised CRP/ESR, connective tissue bloods positive, fibrosis on CXR	Treat underlying cause
Miosis	Drugs- opiates, antipsychotics, cholinergics, nicotine, organophosphates Horner's symptoms, signs of raised ICP (bleed), Argyll-Robertson	Raised drug levels in blood	Antidote if available (e.g. naloxone for opiates)
Mydriasis	CN III lesion – can't close eye, difficulty walking down stairs	Pupil looking down and out, ptosis	Treat underlying tumour –neurosurgical referral
	Drugs – anti-cholinergics, amphetamines	Raised levels of drugs	Antidotes
	Holmes- Adie, physiological, trauma		

Marking Criteria EYE CHANGES	Marks	
	Awarded	Available
Washed hands at the start of the station		1
Introduced themselves – Including First name, last name and role		1
Patient details confirmed: Full name, Age/ D.O.B.		1
Explained purpose of consultation		1
Open question about what brings the patient in today + Clarification of any ambiguity		1
Timeline allows a clear understanding of onset and progression of eye changes - Onset/ Circumstance - Sudden vs. gradual - Fluctuations - Progression - Past episodes		3
Symptoms elicited are relevant and clearly directed at either arriving at a diagnosis or excluding other plausible diagnoses - Sight loss - Pain - Redness - Discharge - Trauma - Glasses		5
Systems queried are relevant to the complaint and adequate questions are asked for each symptom - Neurological; Constitutional		5
Explores **Ideas, Concerns and Expectations**		3
Elicits relevant **Past Medical History** - DM; HTN; Heart problems (esp. AF); Autoimmunity; Cancer		2
Elicits relevant **Drug History** including **Allergies**		2
Elicits relevant **Family History**		2
Elicits relevant **Social History** – including Smoking/ alcohol/ recreational drugs; **Home** environment and support; **Occupation** and impact on life		2
Closes consultation appropriately allowing the patient to ask any questions		1
Presentation: structured, concise		2
Appropriate Differential Diagnosis ± Investigations ± Management Plan		3
Examiner mark – professionalism and rapport		5
Patient mark – professionalism and rapport		5

Consultation	Presentation	Global marks patient	Global marks examiner	Total
$\overline{30}$	$\overline{5}$	$\overline{5}$	$\overline{5}$	$\overline{45}$

75M with decreasing visual acuity in R eye

HPC	1-year history of gradually declining vision. Started as difficulties seeing at night, gradually worsened. Blurry and faded vision now. Decreased acuity of colour vision. Describing halos around lights, especially bright lights. No pain, discharge from eyes, no redness of the eyes and does not feel that the eyes get stuck in the morning. No itching or foreign body sensation reported in eye. Reports no systemic symptoms of infection. no headaches, no head trauma, joint pain, swelling, rash, fever or weight loss reported.
PMHx	HTN, BPH
DHx	Bisoprolol, ramipril, tamsulosin, NKDA
FHx	Brother has early cataract and hypertension
SHx	Lives alone, widowed, self-caring. Looks after grandchildren 3x per week.
ICE	"Doctor, I'm very concerned about this. I need my eyes to look after my grandchildren. My daughter works so I look after the kids. I'll find that very difficult with one eye."
Ix	Ophthalmoscopy.
Dx	Cataract
Tx	Surgery to remove cataract, advise patient that this is very likely to return or affect the other eye

60F with visual disturbance.

HPC	Patient with 4-months history of worsening vision affecting both eyes but right is worse. Says vision deteriorated gradually, describes it as blotchy vision with areas of complete loss of vision. The impairment is independent of light conditions or of time of the day. Reports no eye pain, no sensation of increased ocular pressure. No fever, rash, joint pain, bowel changes, weight loss or night sweats. No discharge from eyes and has not noticed any redness of the eyes. No trauma. No acute life-style changes but has poorly controlled diabetes
PMHx	T1DM diagnosed 25 years ago. HTN
DHx	Insulin, bisoprolol. NKDA
FHx	Nil relevant
SHx	No alcohol, smoking for 35 years. Lives alone. Delivers mail.
ICE	"Doctor, I need my eyesight for my work. I need to drive and read small print address labels. I can't do that anymore. I need to know what's going on, so I can do something about it.
Ix	HbA1c, BM, ophthalmoscopy looking for macular changes (degeneration) and retinopathy.
Dx	Advanced diabetic retinopathy
Tx	Laser surgery, injection of anti-VEGF agent or corticosteroids, vitrectomy, Ophthalmology follow up.

65M with visual disturbances

HPC	Patient with 6-month history of visual field loss. Says this is particularly obvious when driving and he has realized that his peripheral vision is getting worse. One episode of acute and severe eye pain yesterday. patient describes seeing halos around lights. Reports some nausea and vomiting. No headaches. No systemic symptoms of infection. No fever, no abdominal pain, does not feel unsteady and not weak in arms or legs not seeing double either. Does not feel too hot or cold, his bowels are normal. He shaves regularly and his libido is normal. He is not overweight and not complaining of impotence.
PMHx	Migraines, T2DM, HTN
DHx	Ramipril, Metformin, gliclazide, amitriptyline.
FHx	Nil relevant.
SHx	Lives alone, divorced, cab driver. 20 year smoking history. Drinks 3 pints on the weekend.
ICE	"Doctor, do you think this will go away again? I need to be able to drive. I can't pay my bills otherwise."
Ix	Tonometry to determine intraocular pressure, ophthalmoscope to rule out diabetic retinopathy
Dx	Glaucoma.
Tx	Eye drops such as Latanoprost, laser surgery to open blocked drainage tubes or to reduced fluid production, surgery to improve fluid drainage. regular monitoring of intra-ocular pressure.

AUDITORY CHANGES
"WOCH SOCRATES"

<u>**"WIPE"**</u> – Introduce yourself, whilst gaining consent
- Wash hands
- Introduce self – "Hello, my name is X and I am a medical student"
- Patient details – "Could I ask your full name and age?"
- Explain – I have been asked to speak with you about what brings you in, would that be alright?

<u>O</u>pen
- Before we begin can I just ask whether you can hear me well/ if you have a preferred ear or other way for us to communicate?
- I understand you've come in with some hearing problems. Do you mind telling me about that?
- <u>C</u>larification –
- <u>H</u>andedness – "Before asking some more questions about these hearing problems, I'd just like to ask you whether you're left or right handed."

<u>S</u>ite – Does it affect one or both ears?

<u>O</u>nset
1. When did it start? Did anything happen around then?
2. Did it come on suddenly or gradually?
3. Does it come and go or always there?
4. Has it been getting worse?
5. Have you ever had this before?

<u>C</u>haracter
- What kind of sounds do you struggle to hear?
  - ➢ High or low pitch?
  - ➢ Loud noises, whispers?

<u>R</u>adiation
- Is the other ear ever affected?

<u>A</u>ssociated
- Ear – Ask "CAN'T"
  - ➢ **Cleaning** – How do you clean your ears?
  - ➢ **Activities** – Have you gone diving or on a plane recently?
  - ➢ **Noise** – Have you been exposed to high noises?
  - ➢ **Toxicity** – Ask with DHx about ototoxic medication
- Systems
  - ➢ **Ear, Nose, Throat** –
    - ➢ Ear – Pain? Hearing loss? Ringing? Discharge?
    - ➢ Nose – Pain? Bleed? Discharge?
    - ➢ Throat – Pain?
  - ➢ **Neurological** – Headaches? Changes in vision, taste, smell? Weakness? Loss of sensation? Tingling or weird sensations?
  - ➢ **Constitutional** – Any weight loss? Fever? Night-sweats?

<u>T</u>iming – This has been done.

<u>E</u>xacerbating/ relieving
- Does anything make the hearing loss/ ringing/ etc. better or worse?
- Would background noise make a difference?
- Would high versus low pitched noises make a difference?

<u>S</u>everity
- How bad is the hearing loss/ ringing on a scale or 1 -10? 1 being not bothersome at all and 10 being completely impeding you from going about your daily life.

ICE
- You've given me a lot of information, thank you. I'd like to hear a little about what you think could be going on. Do you have any idea?
- Is there anything that's particularly concerning you that you'd like to discuss?
- What exactly are you looking for today, resolution or reassurance?

PMHx
- Do you have any medical conditions?
- Ask a few specific questions to show that you're thinking about different causes
- Specifically, I'd like to ask if you've ever been diagnosed with:
  ➤ Ear problems? Cancer? Chronic illness? High BP? DM? High cholesterol?

DHx
- On any medication? Any doses of medication changed?
- Specifically, ask about "**LACQAA**"
  ➤ Loop diuretics/ Aspirin/ Cytotoxics/ Quinines/ Aminoglycosides/ Alcohol
- Any allergies?

FHx
- Any conditions run in the family?
- Has anyone in the family ever had problems with their hearing?

SHx –
- Smoking/ Alcohol/ Recreational drugs
- Home environment? Support?
- **Occupation** – (Noise exposure in certain occupations!) impact on life and on occupation?

Summarise and Thank
- I'd just like to summarise back to you to make sure I haven't missed anything
- Is there anything you'd like to talk about that we haven't quite addressed?
- Thank you for talking to me and I wish you all the best

Differential Diagnosis

	Diagnosis	Features In History	Features In Investigations	Management
CONDUCTIVE	Otitis media	Fever, ear pain, discharge, recent URTI	Discharge, fluid in middle ear, clouding of tympanic membrane	Antibiotics (drops or oral depending on severity)
	Wax / Foreign Body	Gradual worsening, recurrent, previous wax, use of cotton buds	Wax in ear canal	Warm olive oil, ear syringing
	Others: ➤ **Congenital** ➤ **Otosclerosis** – autosomal dominant so don't miss this in the family history ➤ **Cholesteatoma** – smelly discharge; chronic ear discharge not responding to antibiotics.			
SENSORINEURAL	Tympanic Membrane Rupture	Trauma/ cotton bud use, sudden loss, preceded by ear infection/pain and sudden relief of pain	Ruptured membrane on otoscopy, discharge from ear	Avoid ear drops, tympanoplasty
	Meniere's	Unilateral, full feeling in ear, tinnitus, previous episodes, vertigo	Sensorineural hearing loss with Weber's and Rinne's	Admit if severe symptoms, ENT referral, prochlorperazine for vertigo and N&V
	Others: ➤ **Presbycusis** – especially high frequency usually presents after age of 60 ➤ **Vestibular Schwannoma** - If bilateral, then consider Neurofibromatosis Type II ➤ **Noise-induced damage** – esp. 3-6kHz ➤ **Ototoxic drugs**			

Investigations

Examination	Otoscopy, cranial nerve examination (especially facial and vestibulocochlear), Rinne's and Weber's test, test gait (vestibular)
Bedside	Swab discharge
Bloods	FBC, CRP
Imaging	CT head (cerebellopontine angle)
Special	Audiometry, vestibular evoked responses, nasopharyngoscopy

Marking Criteria AUDITORY CHANGES	Marks	
	Awarded	Available
Washed hands at the start of the station		1
Introduced themselves – Including First name, last name and role		1
Patient details confirmed: Full name, Age/ D.O.B.		1
Explained purpose of consultation		1
Open question about what brings the patient in today + Clarification of any ambiguity		1
Handedness – Briefly enquires about handedness		0
Site – Enquired whether hearing loss affects one ear or both		1
Onset (Timeline) – Asked questions to provide a clear understanding of onset and progression - Onset/ Circumstance - Sudden vs. gradual - Fluctuations - Progression - Past episodes		3
Character - Clarified whether particular sounds are harder to hear		1
Radiation - Ask about the other ear being affected		1
Associated symptoms ▪ **Symptoms** elicited are relevant and clearly directed at either arriving at a diagnosis or excluding other plausible diagnoses – **CAN'T** - Cleaning ears - Activities (diving/ air travel) - Noise - Toxicity (medications/ substances) ▪ **Systems** queried are relevant to the complaint and adequate questions are asked for each symptom - ENT; Neurological; Constitutional		6
Timing - This has been done		0
Exacerbation/ Relief - Clearly asks if the patient has noticed any relieving/ exacerbating factors, providing appropriate examples if prompted (Ex. Background noise)		1
Severity - Subjective quantitative assessment of extent of hearing loss		1
Explores **Ideas, Concerns and Expectations**		3
Elicits relevant **Past Medical History** - Ear problems; cancer; chronic illness; HTN; DM; High cholesterol		2
Elicits relevant **Drug History** including **Allergies**		2
Elicits relevant **Family History**		2
Elicits relevant **Social History** – including Smoking/ alcohol/ recreational drugs; Home environment and support; **Occupation** and impact on life		2
Closes consultation appropriately allowing the patient to ask any questions		1
Presentation: structured, concise		2
Appropriate Differential Diagnosis ± Investigations ± Management Plan		3
Examiner mark – professionalism and rapport		5
Patient mark – professionalism and rapport		5

Consultation	Presentation	Global marks patient	Global marks examiner	Total
30	5	5	5	45

7F with hearing loss.

HPC	Patient with gradually worsening hearing loss. Gradual onset but progressive. Reports significant pain in ear. Fever for 2 days. Noticed that the ear is swollen, red and feels warm to touch. There is no discharge from the ear. Patient complaining of increased salivation and also complaining of pressure sensation in ear. Parents report that the patient has had of sore throat 8 days ago, that was deemed to be viral of nature by the GP. Resolved spontaneously. No foreign travel. Parents say that the patient has recently taken up swimming which she greatly enjoys.
PMHx	Seen for chest infection 3 weeks ago. Otherwise fit and well
DHx	Penicillin allergic (anaphylaxis), nil regular.
FHx	Nil relevant.
SHx	Lives with family. Goes to school. Normal developmental milestones. Vaccinations up to date.
ICE	"Doctor, she's in so much pain and really can't hear from that ear. What can we do to make this go away?"
Ix	FBC, CRP, Otoscopy to inspect tympanic membrane. Consider throat swab for causative pathogens.
Dx	Otitis media.
Tx	Pain relief with paracetamol, NSAIDs, weigh up risk-benefit profile of antibiotics.

70F with gradual hearing loss.

HPC	Patient with 6-months history of unilateral hearing loss. Gradual onset. Affects both ear but right is affected more. No fever, no discharge from the ear. No ringing in the ears. Patient reports no coughs, colds, sore throats or other infections. Feels nauseous and denies any problems on walking, reports no double vision or headaches, visual disturbances or balance problems. Reports some feeling of tightness and tenderness in her jaw when chewing and feels like she can hear her jaw joint "pop" which she never used to before. Finds herself chewing more on the other side as it is less uncomfortable.
PMHx	HTN, Asthma
DHx	Bisoprolol, ramipril, amlodipine, salbutamol inhaler
FHx	Father died age 60 from stroke.
ICE	"Doctor, is this normal for my age or is there something wrong? I always thought when you get older, you get harder of hearing, but my right is much worse than my left."
Ix	Otoscopy to investigate auditory canal for obstruction.
Dx	Obstruction of auditory canal with wax
Tx	Olive oil ear drops or hydrogen peroxide ear drops, severe cases may require syringing

60M with gradual hearing loss and impaired balance

HPC	Patient with increasing hearing loss over 5 years. Significant progress over last 2 months. He has also noticed ringing in his left ear. Patient also describes problems with balance. Reports no headaches, no SOB or chest pain. No head trauma. He denies any behaviour or personality changes or cognitive decline. There is no weakness, speech changes, swallowing difficulties or double vision. He has been fully independent and mobile but has noticed that he is getting slightly unsteady on his feet and feels dizzy. He feels his face is weird to touch and appears a bit lopsided.
PMHx	Nil. Fit and healthy.
DHx	Nil regular. Occasional paracetamol PRN.
FHx	Diabetes and heart disease on father's side.
SHx	Lives with wife, no children. Works at Tesco. Non-smoker. No alcohol. Ex-alcoholic.
ICE	"I have been doing some reading and, on the internet, it says that I could have a brain tumour. Or maybe a stroke. That would explain the paralysis on one side of my face. What do you think, doctor?"
Ix	FBC, LFT, U&E, lipid profile, glucose, HbA1C, Otoscopy to exclude ocular pathology, CT head, consider MRI head.
Dx	Acoustic neuroma.
Tx	Surgical removal or radiotherapy, depending on risk profile. Advise patient of possible complications associated with nerve damage. Physiotherapy for unsteadiness, hearing aids.

DIZZINESS & VERTIGO
GENERAL FRAMEWORK

"**W**IPE" – Introduce yourself, whilst gaining consent
- Wash hands
- Introduce self – "Hello, my name is X and I am a medical student"
- Patient details – "Could I ask your full name and age?"
- Explain – I have been asked to speak with you about what brings you in, would that be alright?

Open
- I understand you've been feeling dizzy, could you tell me about that?
- **Clarify** – I would just like to clarify what you mean when you say dizzy. Do you mean you feel like you're about to faint or that the room is spinning around?
- **Handedness** – "Before asking some more questions about this dizziness I'd just like to ask you whether you're left or right handed."

Timeline
1. When did this start? Did anything happen around then?
2. Did it start suddenly or gradually?
3. Does this dizziness come and go or is it always there?
4. Has this dizziness been getting worse?
5. Have you ever had this dizziness before?

Symptoms
- **TIP**
    - ➤ **Trauma** – Have you had any recent trauma or impacts to the head?
    - ➤ **Infection** – Have you been ill recently?
    - ➤ **Position** – Does position make any difference to the dizziness?
- **Ears**
    - ➤ **Deafness** – Has your hearing been affected at all?
    - ➤ **Tinnitus** – Have you experienced any ringing in your ear?
    - ➤ **Discharge** – Have you noticed any discharge from your ears?
    - ➤ **Fullness** – Have you experienced any fullness in your ear?
- **Relieving/ Exacerbating factors**
    - ➤ MUST ask about head turning for BPPV, any relationship to change in posture

Systems
- **Neurological** – Have you had a headache? Noticed a change in any of your senses? And what about any weakness or altered sensation?
- **Ear, Nose, Throat** –
    - ➤ Ear – Pain? Hearing loss? Ringing? Discharge?
    - ➤ Nose – Pain? Bleed? Discharge?
    - ➤ Throat – Pain?
- Dermatological – Any skin changes? Any rashes? Any ulcers (Esp. around ear – Ramsay Hunt)
- **Cardiovascular** – Any heart problems? Any palpitations (esp. when dizzy/ light-headed)? Any SOB?
- **Constitutional** – Have you felt tired? Loss of appetite? Weight loss?

ICE
- You've given me a lot of information, thank you. I'd like to hear a little about what you think could be going on. Do you have any idea?
- Is there anything that's particularly concerning you that you'd like to discuss?
- What exactly are you looking for today, resolution or reassurance?

PMHx
- Do you have any medical conditions?
- Ask a few specific questions to show that you're thinking about different causes
- Specifically, I'd like to ask if you've ever had:
  - ➤ A stroke or something called a transient ischaemic attack? Diabetes? High blood pressure? High cholesterol? Any ear problems? Migraine?

PMHx
- Any medical conditions?
  - ➤ Previous stroke? Recent trauma?

DHx
- On any medication? Any doses of medication changed?
- Specifically, ask about "**LACQAA**"
  - ➤ Loop diuretics/ Aspirin/ Cytotoxics/ Quinines/ Aminoglycosides/ Alcohol
- Any allergies?

FHx
- Any conditions run in the family? Specifically, any diabetes? High BP? High cholesterol? Multiple sclerosis?
- Has anyone in the family ever had problems with dizziness similar to the one you're experiencing now?

SHx –
- Smoking/ Alcohol/ Recreational drugs
- Home environment? Support?
- Occupation – impact on life and on occupation?

Summarise and Thank
- I'd just like to summarise back to you to make sure I haven't missed anything
- Is there anything you'd like to talk about that we haven't quite addressed?
- Thank you for talking to me and I wish you all the best

Differential Diagnosis

	Diagnosis	Features In History	Features In Investigations	Management
PERIPHERAL	**Benign Paroxysmal Positional Vertigo**	Extreme vertigo on changing position (e.g. in bed), settles if they stay still, room spins, no LOC	Positive Dix-Hallpike	Epley's manoeuvre, anti-emetics. Prochlorperazine
	Viral labyrinthitis	Fever/prodromal URTI, ear pain		Symptomatic management
CENTRAL	**Stroke / TIA**	Sudden onset dizziness / vertigo, associated unilateral weakness/ numbness	Unilateral nystagmus, unsteady gait, unilateral weakness and reduced sensation, positive Babinski	CT head, consider thrombolysis if within 4h of onset, admit under stroke team
	Ototoxicity	History of ototoxic drugs, gradual onset and worsening	Reduced hearing on audiometry	Cease ototoxic medication, rehabilitate
	Postural Hypotension	Dizzy when patients stands up	Postural BP Drop of >20 mmHg Systolic	Rehydrate, reducing diuretic dose, fludrocortisone

Investigations

	General	Specific
Examination	Full neurological examination incl. cranial nerves (?nystagmus), otoscopy, gait analysis	
Bedside	Dix-Hallpike manoeuvre, lying and standing BP,	
Bloods	FBC, CRP, U&E	Stroke: coagulation screen
Imaging	CT head	
Special	Audiometry	MS: lumbar puncture, MRI head and spine

Marking Criteria DIZZINESS	Marks	
	Awarded	Available
Washed hands at the start of the station		1
Introduced themselves – Including First name, last name and role		1
Patient details confirmed: Full name, Age/ D.O.B.		1
Explained purpose of consultation		1
Open question about what brings the patient in today + Clarification of any ambiguity – E.g. Feeling faint vs. room spinning		1
Handedness – Briefly enquires about handedness		0
Timeline allows a clear understanding of onset and progression - Onset/ Circumstance - Sudden vs. gradual - Fluctuations - Progression - Past episodes		3

Symptoms elicited are relevant and clearly directed at either arriving at a diagnosis or excluding other plausible diagnoses
    o "TIP"
      ▪ Trauma
      ▪ Infection
      ▪ Position
    o Ears
      ▪ Deafness
      ▪ Tinnitus
      ▪ Discharge
      ▪ Ear fullness
    o Exacerbating/ Reliving factors
      ▪ Specifically head turning
		5

Systems queried are relevant to the complaint and adequate questions are asked for each symptom - Neurological; ENT; Cardiovascular; Dermatological; Constitutional		5
Explores **Ideas, Concerns and Expectations**		3
Elicits relevant **Past Medical History** - Past stroke or TIA; DM; HTN; High cholesterol; Ear problems generally; Migraine		2
Elicits relevant **Drug History** including **Allergies**		2
Elicits relevant **Family History**		2
Elicits relevant **Social History** – including Smoking/ alcohol/ recreational drugs; **H**ome environment and support; **O**ccupation and impact on life		2
Closes consultation appropriately allowing the patient to ask any questions		1
Presentation: structured, concise		2
Appropriate Differential Diagnosis ± Investigations ± Management Plan		3
Examiner mark – professionalism and rapport		5
Patient mark – professionalism and rapport		5

Consultation	Presentation	Global marks patient	Global marks examiner	Total
$\overline{30}$	$\overline{5}$	$\overline{5}$	$\overline{5}$	$\overline{45}$

55M presenting with dizziness and vertigo when standing.

HPC	Patient reports 6-months history of sudden onset of vertigo. This is triggered by movement, especially head turning. No ringing in the ears and no hearing loss. No vertigo at rest or when sitting still. It was noticeable occasionally before but now, even turning in bed brings on symptoms. Patient reports no systemic symptoms of infection. No fever, no headaches, no palpitations, no SOB, no CP. No head trauma. No unsteadiness, no persistent dizzy spells, vertigo, no weakness, denies feeling different, swallowing problems, double vision. He has noticed that when he has these episodes, "he is unable to read and everything is jumpy."
PMHx	Chest infection 4 weeks ago, given antibiotics. Nil chronic.
DHx	Multivitamins, paracetamol PRN, nil regular. NKDA
FHx	Nil relevant.
SHx	Lives alone. Businessman. Social drinking. No smoking. No IVDU.
ICE	"Doctor, this is becoming unbearable. I'm trying not to move my head to I don't get dizzy, but now I'm all stiff and sore in my neck."
Ix	FBC, U&E, LFT, Otoscopy, Dix-Hallpike test, Rarely, imaging CT head required to reassure/rule out sinister cause.
Dx	Benign positional vertigo
Tx	Usually self-resolving, consider decreasing alcohol intake, betahistine or cochlear sedatives such as prochlorperazine.

32M with vertigo

HPC	Patient presents with sudden onset vertigo for the past 7 hours. This started suddenly without warning. He has had several similar episodes over the past 6 months, most resolving within 24 hours. Complains of nausea and vomiting as well as ringing in both ears. He is also struggling to hear at times and feels a pressure like sensation in both ears. He has not noticed any discharge from the ears. He does not feel unsteady and has not noticed any weakness of limbs. There is no swallowing problem or speech changes. He has not noticed any diplopia. Denies fever or other systemic signs of infection. No LOC, headache or seizures. No head trauma.
PMHx	Nil. Fit and well.
DHx	NKDA.
FHx	Father diagnosed with lung cancer age 84, mother T1DM
SHx	Works as pilot. No alcohol or smoking. No IVDU.
ICE	"Doctor, I need these attacks to stop. I can't work like this. I'm putting my passengers at risk if I fly in this condition."
Ix	FBC, U&E, LFT, MRI brain, hearing tests (Audiometry)
Dx	Ménière's disease
Tx	Betahistine, Prochlorpromazine, surgery to insert Endo lymphatic shunts

25M with sudden onset vertigo

HPC	Patient with sudden onset vertigo. This started suddenly and is gradually getting worse for last few hours. Complaining of nausea and vomiting. Symptoms worsened by head movements. No tinnitus or discharge from ears. He has not noticed any deafness or changes in his hearing. Reports acute viral chest infection with fever the previous week. Chest infection resolving. No ataxia, no headache, no loss of consciousness, no neurological symptoms, no swallowing/speech problems. No systemic symptoms of infection. Generally fit and well. Exercises regularly. Not obese.
PMHx	Nil chronic, chest infection 1 week ago. HSV 1 infection, facial cold sores.
DHx	Nil regular. Paracetamol during chest infection. NKDA
FHx	Nil relevant
ICE	"This feels terrible, doctor. The room feels like its spinning and it just won't stop. I'm nauseous all the time. I need something for that. I constantly feel like I'm going to vomit. Can't keep any food down."
Ix	FBC, CRP, LFT, U&E, CT head, otoscopy to rule out otitis media
Dx	Acute vestibular failure
Tx	Usually spontaneously improves over days, fully resolves over course of weeks, consider cyclizine or Methylprednisolone to improve patient's quality of life.

FITS, FALLS AND FUNNY TURNS
UNIQUE STRUCTURE - BASED ON A DETAILED TIMELINE OF EVENTS

<u>**"WIPE"**</u> – Introduce yourself, whilst gaining consent
- Wash hands
- Introduce self – "Hello, my name is X and I am a medical student"
- Patient details – "Could I ask your full name and age?"
- Explain – I have been asked to speak with you about what brings you in, would that be alright?

<u>**Open**</u>
- **Open** – I'm sorry to hear that you've had a fall, would you mind telling me about what happened?
- **Clarify** – Can I just clarify how you fell? Did you faint, lose balance, trip?
- **Handedness** - "Before asking some more questions about the fall, I'd just like to ask you whether you're left or right handed."

<u>**TIMELINE & SYMPTOMS**</u>
(2, 5, 5, 2)
- **Before**
    1. **Feeling** – What did you **feel** immediately before the episode?
    2. **Warning** – Did you **realise** you were about to fall?
- **During**
    1. **LOC** – During the fall did you lose consciousness?
        a. **Duration** – (If yes) How long were you out for?
    2. **Witness** – Did anyone see what happened?
        a. **Movements** – (If yes) Did they say anything about any movements?
    3. **Incontinence** – A more personal question. Were you incontinent of urine or faeces?
    4. **Tongue** – Did you bite your tongue?
    5. **Injuries** – Did you hit your head? Injure yourself?
- **After**
    1. **Feeling** – **How** did you feel immediately after the fall?
    2. **Amnesia** – Could you **remember** what happened?
    3. **Todd's paresis** – Did you feel **weak** afterwards?
    4. **Muscle pain** – Did your muscles **ache** afterwards?
    5. **Confusion/ sleepiness** – Did you feel **drowsy**?
- **Finish timeline**
    1. Is this the first time this has happened?
    2. (If not) Is it becoming increasingly frequent?

Systems
- **Cardiovascular** – Did you have any chest pain? Palpitations? SOB? Do you feel breathless lying down or at night? Do you prop yourself up with pillows? Do you often get ankle/ lower back swelling? Any cough (blood in sputum),
- **Neurological** – Any headaches? Change sight, smell, taste, hearing? Weakness? Weird sensation anywhere in your body?
- **Leg pain/swelling, travel history, risk factors for thromboembolic disease (smoking, past/family history, long travel within 6 weeks, immobilisations, recent surgery)**

<u>**ICE**</u>
- You've given me a lot of information, thank you. I'd like to hear a little about what you think could be going on. Do you have any idea?
- Is there anything that's particularly concerning you that you'd like to discuss?
- What exactly are you looking for today, resolution or reassurance?

PMHx
- Do you have any medical conditions?
- Ask a few specific questions to show that you're thinking about different causes
- Specifically, I'd like to ask if you've ever been diagnosed with:
  - ➤ Epilepsy? Low BP? Heart problems? Sight problems? Mobility issues?

DHx
- On any medication? Any doses of medication changed?
  - ➤ (Polypharmacy is an independent risk factor for falls) Specifically ask about: BP medication, sedatives, osteoporosis medication
- Any allergies?

FHx
- Any conditions run in the family? Specifically, epilepsy?
- Has anyone in the family ever had problems with falls?
  - ➤ Epilepsy? Heart problems? Any FHx of **sudden death**? Clots in the legs or lungs?

SHx –
- Smoking/ Alcohol/ Recreational drugs
- Home environment? Support?
- Occupation – impact on life and on occupation?

CONSENT FOR COLLATERAL history – For the team to get a good picture of exactly what happened, it would be useful for us to talk to whoever witnessed your fall, would that be possible/ okay with you?

Summarise and Thank
- I'd just like to summarise back to you to make sure I haven't missed anything
- Is there anything you'd like to talk about that we haven't quite addressed?
- Thank you for talking to me and I wish you all the best

Investigations

Examination	Cardiac - ?murmur Neurological – weakness / reduced proprioception / sensation Fundoscopy - ?raised ICP General – signs of dehydration (tachycardic, low BP, dry mucous membranes, low JVP)
Bedside	Lying and standing blood pressures, ECG (?Silent MI), urine dip
Bloods	FBC, CRP, U&E, lactate, troponin
Imaging	CXR, CT head,
Special	EEG, echocardiogram, 24 hour Holter monitor, tilt table test

Differential Diagnosis

	Diagnosis	Features In History	Features In Investigations	Management
NEUROGENIC	**Vasovagal**	Before: Lightheaded / flushed before, hot place, standing for a long time During: brief LOC (<1min), no features of seizure (rarely: incontinence and twitches) After: quick recovery, not post ictal, not flushed	Nil findings on investigations	Reassurance
	Seizure	Before: Aura, trigger (lights / alcohol), previous history of seizure, decreased anti-epileptic During: LOC, incontinence, lateral tongue biting, twitches, eyes rolled, unresponsive After: slow recovery (hours), initial confusion	Raised lactate post ictal CT head may reveal source (injury / tumour) in secondary seizure	Anti-epileptics if not first event, neurology follow up
CARDIOGENIC	**Postural hypotension**	Before: Just sat or stood up, felt suddenly light headed, blackness of vision During: No features of seizure, brief LOC After: Quick recovery, not post ictal	Drop in BP on standing, with tachycardia Dehydration on examination, raised urea on bloods	Rehydrate, consider reducing diuretic dose, fludrocortisone
	Aortic stenosis	Before: Exertional chest pain and light headedness. During: Brief LOC, no seizure activity After: Quick recovery, no symptoms at rest	Ejection systolic murmur on examination, slow rising pulse, low pulse pressure Diagnosed on echocardiogram for severity	Cardiology follow up for a possible valvuloplasty or replacement
	Arrhythmia	Before: Palpitations, drug over dose, chest pain, lightheaded During: Brief LOC, no seizure activity, pale looking After: flushed afterwards, quick recovery	ECG may show arrhythmia (e.g. AF) or long QT (predisposes to arrhythmia, possibly due to drugs) Drug levels in blood may be high, abnormal electrolytes on bloods	Cardiac monitoring Anti-dote for overdoses Cardiology follow up if persistent rhythm

Also consider: ACS, PE, mechanical fall, Alcohol intoxication

Marking Criteria FITS/ FAINTS	Marks	
	Awarded	Available
Washed hands at the start of the station		1
Introduced themselves – Including First name, last name and role		1
Patient details confirmed: Full name, Age/ D.O.B.		1
Explained purpose of consultation		1
Open question about what brings the patient in today + Clarification of any ambiguity – E.g. Tiredness vs. malaise (if unclear)		1
Handedness – Briefly enquires about handedness		0

Timeline – very detailed timeline broken up into before; during; after; missing questions
 - **Before**
     o Feeling; Warning
 - **During**
     o LOC; Duration; Witness; Movements; Incontinence; Tongue; Injuries
 - **After**
     o Feeling; Amnesia; Paresis; Pain; Confusion/ sleepiness
 - **Finish timeline**
     o Previous episodes? If so, increasing frequency?
		8

Systems queried are relevant to the complaint and adequate questions are asked for each symptom - Neurological; Cardiovascular		5
Explores **Ideas, Concerns and Expectations**		3
Elicits relevant **Past Medical History** - Epilepsy; Low BP; Heart problems; Sight problems; Mobility issues		2
Elicits relevant **Drug History** including **Allergies**		2
Elicits relevant **Family History**		2
Elicits relevant **Social History** – including Smoking/ alcohol/ recreational drugs; **Home** environment and support; **Occupation** and impact on life		2
Closes consultation appropriately allowing the patient to ask any questions		1
Presentation: structured, concise		2
Appropriate Differential Diagnosis ± Investigations ± Management Plan		3
Examiner mark – professionalism and rapport		5
Patient mark – professionalism and rapport		5

Consultation	Presentation	Global marks patient	Global marks examiner	Total
30	5	5	5	45

70F with recurring faints

HPC	Patient presenting with 1-year history of recurring faints and blackouts. Reports several falls associated with blackouts. During blackouts, which are never more than few seconds, he is able to hear and see things around him. The episodes are triggered by getting up quickly and are worse after sleeping. He feels slightly dizzy and that his heart is racing just before the fall. He has not noticed any twitching or bladder/bowel incontinence during these episodes. No headaches, no dizziness, no tinnitus, no head trauma, no infective symptoms. No ataxia, swallowing or speech problems. Denies palpitations. No CP/SOB/hearing loss/ringing in the ears. This started after his visit to the GP when his BP was high.
PMHx	HTN, T2DM - diet controlled, newly diagnosed AF
DHx	Bisoprolol, Amlodipine, Ramipril, Warfarin
FHx	Nil relevant.
SHx	Independent. Lives alone. Three times a week POC to help with shopping. Occasional alcohol. Non-smoker.
ICE	"Doctor, I'm just so worried that I'm going to pass out and fall and hit my head. I'm on that new medication you know. I need to get all these blood tests done and the GP says I need to be very careful that I don't cut myself because I will bleed a lot. What if I hit my head and cut it?"
Ix	FBC, LFT, U&E, TFT, lying and standing BP
Dx	Postural hypotension
Tx	Adjust BP medication. If AF is new, heart efficiency is reduced. Addition of bisoprolol for rate control will lower HR and delay/reduce sympathetic response to drop in BP. Physiotherapy

20M with recurring fits

HPC	Brought to the hospital having had a fit at home. Has had recurring fits in the past. Significant sweating and anxiety. Feels very agitated and restless. Has had few fits previously which resolves spontaneously. He feels his hands are very shaky and he has been nauseous and vomiting non-stop. No obvious source of bleeding. No PR bleeding, no haematemesis. No fever, rash, headache, chest pain or neurological defect or trauma. No ataxia. Oriented and alert. Not drowsy. Says he feels like his skin is itching and crawling with bugs. Denies and IV drug use.
PMHx	Nil.
DHx	NKDA. Nil regular.
FHx	Nil regular.
SHx	Lives with girlfriend. Non-smoker. 30 units per day alcohol, but completely quit 4 days ago.
ICE	"Doctor, my girlfriend is going to leave me. I'm trying to stop, but it's so hard!"
Ix	FBC, LFTs, U&E, Amylase, Vitamin B, CT head (if head injury or confused)
Dx	Acute severe alcohol withdrawal.
Tx	Fluid resuscitation, chlordiazepoxide in appropriate dosing as per local guidelines. Regular and PRN. Pabrinex, drinking cessation advice, Advise not to drive, admit until stable.

70F with acute collapse

HPC	Sudden collapse, witnessed by daughter. Now rousable, but very drowsy. No head trauma. Reports no SOB or chest pain. Reports feeling dizzy and reports that "the world is spinning". No Headache. No tongue biting, no incontinence, no limb jerking. Appears acutely confused. Fever for last 2 days. Also having severe diarrhoea and vomiting in the last week with no oral intake for 5 days. No blood in stool or mucus. Has been feeling very tired and exhausted. Unable to sit up due to pain. Shallow breathing, struggling to complete sentences.
PMHx	Hip fracture 2 years ago. Osteoporosis, arthritis in knees. Diverticulitis.
DHx	Adcal D3, alendronic acid, Simvastatin, NKDA
SHx	Lives with daughter and son in law. Retired. No alcohol or smoking.
ICE	"Doctor, What am I doing here? Who are all these people? I don't think I'm supposed to be here."
Ix	U&E, glucose, LFT, coagulation screen, blood cultures, FBC, CRP, stool sample (microscopy/culture).
Dx	Septic shock
Tx	Sepsis 6 - Empirical Antibiotics until cultures back, fluid resuscitation, paracetamol, Catheterise

WEAKNESS
"WOCH SOCRATES"

WIPE" – Introduce yourself, whilst gaining consent
- Wash hands
- Introduce self – "Hello, my name is X and I am a medical student"
- Patient details – "Could I ask your full name and age?"
- Explain – "I have been asked to speak with you about what brings you in, would that be alright?"

Open
- I understand you've been experiencing some weakness, can you tell me more about that?
- **C**larification
- **H**andedness – "Before asking some more questions about the fall, I'd just like to ask you whether you're left or right handed."

Site – Where exactly is the weakness?

Onset
1. When did this weakness start?
2. Did it come on suddenly or gradually?
3. Does the weakness come and go or is it always there?
4. Has the weakness been getting worse?
5. Have you ever had weakness like this before?

Character – Can you describe the weakness? Is it weak from the start or do you mean that it tires quickly?

Radiation – Does the weakness affect any other parts of your body?

Associated
- Symptoms
  - ➢ **Sensation** – Is this weakness associated with a loss of **sensation**?
  - ➢ **Pain** – Is this weakness associated with **pain**?
  - ➢ **Wasting** – Have you noticed a **wasting** of the affected muscles?
  - ➢ **Stiffness** – Is the weakness associated with **stiffness** of the muscles?
  - ➢ **Twitching** – Have you noticed any **twitching** of the muscles?

  - ➢ **Eyes** – Have you noticed a **drooping** of the eyes? Difficult **eye movement**?
  - ➢ **Sphincter control** – More personal question. Have you been **incontinent** of urine or faeces?
- Systems
  - ➢ **Neurological** – Any headaches? A change in any of your senses? Weakness? Weird sensation anywhere in your body?
  - ➢ **Musculoskeletal** – Any back or joint pain? Any stiffness?
  - ➢ **Dermatological** – Any skin changes? Rashes? Ulcers?
  - ➢ **Constitutional** – Have you felt tired? Loss of appetite? Weight loss?

Timing – This has been done.

Exacerbating/ relieving
- Does anything make the weakness better or worse?
  - ➢ Exercise/ rest?
  - ➢ Heating/ cooling?

Severity – How bad is weakness? Try to rate according to MRC Grade if you have the time. (See below)

ICE
- You've given me a lot of information, thank you. I'd like to hear a little about what you think could be going on. Do you have any idea?
- Is there anything that's particularly concerning you that you'd like to discuss?
- What exactly are you looking for today, resolution or reassurance?

PMHx
- Do you have any medical conditions?
- Ask a few specific questions to show that you're thinking about different causes
- Specifically, I'd like to ask if you've ever been diagnosed with:
  - ➢ Diabetes? Cancer? Muscle disease? Slipped disc? Stroke or something called a transient ischaemic attack?

DHx
- On any medication? Any doses of medication changed?
- Any allergies?

FHx
- Any conditions run in the family? Specifically, I'd like to ask about muscle conditions? Nervous system conditions? Something called an autoimmune condition?
- Has anyone in the family ever been affected by a weakness similar to the one you're describing to me now?

SHx –
- **S**moking/ Alcohol/ Recreational drugs
- **H**ome environment? Support?
- **O**ccupation – impact on life and on occupation?

Summarise and Thank
- I'd just like to summarise back to you to make sure I haven't missed anything
- Is there anything you'd like to talk about that we haven't quite addressed?

Thank you for talking to me and I wish you all the best

Differential Diagnosis

Diagnosis	Features In History	Features In Investigations	Management
Myasthenia Gravis	Worse at the end of the day, difficulty swallowing at end of meal, voice gets softer, ptosis, diplopia	Fatiguability, ice test for ptosis, bloods (anti-AChR, anti- MUSK, anti-LRP), (tensilon test)	CT chest ?thymoma Pyridostygmine, immunosuppression Neurology follow up,
Lambert-Eaton Myaesthenic Syndrome	Gradual onset weakness (legs > arms), fatigue on exercise, autonomic (dry mouth, constipation)	Decreased reflexes, improvement of strength with repetition (opposite of MG),	Look for tumour as majority associated with cancer (most SCC lung), Immunosuppression if no cancer.
Guillain–Barré	Progressive bilateral weakness, ascending from lower limbs, 4-6 weeks after diarrhoeal illness in previously fit, few sensation changes (NB Miller Fischer is a variant that bilaterally progresses descending from the head)	Reduced / absent reflexes, hypotonic Raised CSF protein and no raised CSF cell counts	IV Ig, plasmapheresis, Spirometry for FVC (risk of respiratory failure – ICU needed), ECG for heart block, neurology input
Multiple Sclerosis	Weakness, non-anatomical distribution, worse weakness with heat (after hot bath). History of neurological symptoms separated in space and time	MRI brain and spine shows demyelinating lesions correlating to neurological symptoms.	Neurology input Immunosuppression

Investigations

Examination	Full neurological examination incl. cranial nerves and tests of fatigability
Bedside	Urine dip, lying and standing blood pressure
Bloods	FBG, U&E, LFTs, CRP, ESR TFTs (hypothyroid weakness), bone profile (hypocalcaemia), Vitamin B12 and folate (peripheral neuropathies), HbA1c (peripheral neuropathy in poor diabetes control)
Imaging	CT and MRI head and spinal cord, CXR (?thymic shadow)
Special	Nerve conduction studies, electromyography

Marking Criteria WEAKNESS	Marks	
	Awarded	Available
Washed hands at the start of the station		1
Introduced themselves – Including First name, last name and role		1
Patient details confirmed: Full name, Age/ D.O.B.		1
Explained purpose of consultation		1
Open question about what brings the patient in today + Clarification of any ambiguity		1
Handedness – Briefly enquires about handedness		0
Site – Enquired about exact location of weakness		1
Onset (Timeline) – Asked questions to provide a clear understanding of onset and progression - Onset/ Circumstance - Sudden vs. gradual - Fluctuations - Progression - Past episodes		3
Character - Clarified weakness – Ex. Weakness throughout vs. tires quickly		1
Radiation - Asked about weakness in other regions of body		1
Associated symptoms ▪ **Symptoms** elicited are relevant and clearly directed at either arriving at a diagnosis or excluding other plausible diagnoses - Sensation; Pain; Stiffness; Wasting; Twitching - Eyes; Sphincter control ▪ **Systems** queried are relevant to the complaint and adequate questions are asked for each symptom - Neurological; Musculoskeletal; Dermatological; Constitutional		6
Timing - This has been done		0
Exacerbation/ Relief - Clearly asks if the patient has noticed any relieving/ exacerbating factors, providing appropriate examples if prompted (Ex. Exercise/ rest; heating/ cooling)		1
Severity - Subjective quantitative assessment of extent of weakness - Best candidates may attempt to quantify objectively determining the MRC Grade		1
Explores **Ideas, Concerns and Expectations**		3
Elicits relevant **Past Medical History** - DM; Cancer; Muscle disease; Slipped disc; Prior stroke or TIA		2
Elicits relevant **Drug History** including **Allergies**		2
Elicits relevant **Family History**		2
Elicits relevant **Social History** – including Smoking/ alcohol/ recreational drugs; Home environment and support; Occupation and impact on life		2
Closes consultation appropriately allowing the patient to ask any questions		1
Presentation: structured, concise		2
Appropriate Differential Diagnosis ± Investigations ± Management Plan		3
Examiner mark – professionalism and rapport		5
Patient mark – professionalism and rapport		5

Consultation	Presentation	Global marks patient	Global marks examiner	Total
30	5	5	5	45

60M with acute onset left sided weakness.

HPC	Found by wife in bed, unable to move arms or legs on left side. Slurred speech and facial droop. Alert and responsive. Wife reports that he can hold a normal conversation and has not noticed headache, fall, head injury, swallowing problems. Denies any visual problems or double vision or nystagmus. No chest pain, no SOB, no systemic features of infection. No ataxia or tinnitus. No discharge from ears or nose. No dizziness or vertigo. No pain in limbs or back. Normal sensation and power on the right.
PMHx	HTN, heart disease, 3x CABG
DHx	Aspirin, simvastatin bisoprolol, NKDA
SHx	Ex-smoker. Alcohol intake of 10 units per day, builder.
ICE	"Doctor, is there any chance this is going to improve? Will I ever walk again?"
Ix	FBC, U&E, LFT, glucose, coagulation screen, Lipids, ECG, CT/MRI brain, carotid Doppler
Dx	Stroke, right hemisphere.
Tx	Depends on result of imaging. If haemorrhage, neurosurgical advice re: evacuation of Haematoma. Not for thrombolysis at this point as time of onset unknown but should be managed in HASU (ideally) Consider anticoagulation with enoxaparin and clopidogrel. If AF, anticoagulation. Physiotherapy/rehabilitation.

45F with episodes of weakness

HPC	Patient reports several episodes for weakness and paraesthesia. Also complaining of double vision and fatigue. Feels unsteady on walking and tends to fall. Has become constipated despite unaltered eating habits. Reports muscle spasms and feels very anxious. No headaches, no chest pain, no muscle pain. Feels stiff. No ataxia or tinnitus. No discharge from ears or nose. No dizziness or vertigo. Reports no trauma to head or limbs. No infective symptoms. Oriented in time, place and person. No confusion. No loss of consciousness. No slurred speech or facial droop. No incontinence or seizures.
PMHx	T1DM
DHx	NKDA, Insulin.
FHx	Mother had Grave's disease.
SHx	Independent. Fit and well. Drinks socially. No smoking history.
ICE	"Doctor, I'm very worried about what is going on. I've been having these episodes when I can't move and get so tired and lethargic and I feel like they have only been getting worse. I don't know what to do anymore."
Ix	MRI brain, lumbar puncture testing for evidence of chronic inflammation, oligoclonal bands.
Dx	Multiple sclerosis.
Tx	Supportive. Counselling. Lifestyle advice. Encourage exercise. Interferon therapy, methyl prednisolone pulsed therapy for acute episode, MS nurse and counselling

85M with weakness

HPC	Patient with 1-week episode of vomiting and poor oral intake presents with global weakness. He recently was admitted to the hospital after a severe episode of diarrhoea and made good recovery but his symptoms have returned. Complaining of leg cramps and constipation. Weakness is non-specific affecting whole of the body. He feels that he does not have to the energy to do anything and feel very exhausted. No headaches and does not feel unsteady, confused, speech or swallowing problems. No pain in abdomen or distension. Does not feel sore anywhere.
PMHx	HTN, Heart failure
DHx	Bisoprolol, furosemide. NKDA
SHx	Non-smoker. Lives alone at home. Widowed. Self-caring. Smokes pipes.
FHx	Nil relevant.
ICE	"Doctor, I didn't really think much of this all, but now I'm not able to walk my dog anymore. I just can't lift her up when we walk up the stairs to the house."
Ix	Assess fluid status, FBC, U&E, LFT
Dx	Hypokalaemia secondary to vomiting and diuretic use.
Tx	Fluid resuscitation. Potassium replacement, suspend furosemide, start on potassium sparing diuretic, symptom control

ALTERED SENSATION
"WOCH SOCRATES"

"**W**IPE" – Introduce yourself, whilst gaining consent
- Wash hands
- Introduce self – "Hello, my name is X and I am a medical student"
- Patient details – "Could I ask your full name and age?"
- Explain – "I have been asked to speak with you about what brings you in, would that be alright?"

Open
- I understand you've been experiencing some odd feelings in your body, can you tell me more about that?
- **C**larification
- **H**andedness – "Before asking some more questions about the fall, I'd just like to ask you whether you're left or right handed."

Site
- Where exactly are you feeling these sensations?

Onset
1. When did the sensation start? What were you doing then?
2. Did the sensation come on suddenly or gradually?
3. Does the sensation come and go or is it always there?
4. Has the sensation been getting worse?
5. Have you ever had a sensation like this before?

Character
- Can you describe exactly what the sensation feels like?

Radiation
- Do you feel this anywhere else?

Associated
- Symptoms
  - ➤ (If PC pins & needles) **Numbness** – Do you have any numbness?
  - ➤ (If PC numbness) **Pins & Needles** – Do you have any pins & needles?

  - ➤ **Weakness**– Is this sensation associated with weakness of the muscles?
  - ➤ **Pain** – Is this sensation associated with pain?
  - ➤ **Wasting** – Have you noticed wasting of the affected muscles?
  - ➤ **Stiffness** – Is the weakness associated with stiffness of the muscles?
  - ➤ **Twitching** – Have you noticed any twitching of the muscles?

  - ➤ **Eyes** – Have you noticed drooping of the eyes? Difficult eye movement?
  - ➤ **Sphincter control** – A more personal question. Have you been incontinent of urine or faeces recently?

- Systems
  - ➤ **Neurological** – Any headaches? A change in any of your senses? Weakness?
  - ➤ **Anxiety** – Would you consider yourself an anxious person? Do you think it could be related?
  - ➤ **Constitutional** – Have you felt tired? Loss of appetite? Weight loss?

Timing – This has been done.

Exacerbating/ Relieving factors
- Does anything make the numbness worse?
  - ➤ Exercise/ rest?
  - ➤ Heating/ cooling?
  - ➤ Anxiety?

Severity – How bad is this sensation, from 1 to 10? 1 being not bothersome and 10 being impeding you from carrying out your daily activities.

ICE
- You've given me a lot of information, thank you. I'd like to hear a little about what you think could be going on. Do you have any idea?
- Is there anything that's particularly concerning you that you'd like to discuss?
- What exactly are you looking for today, resolution or reassurance?

PMHx
- Do you have any medical conditions?
- Ask a few specific questions to show that you're thinking about different causes
  - ➤ Specifically, I'd like to ask if you've ever been diagnosed with
    Diabetes? High BP? High cholesterol? Nervous system diseases? Spinal cord problems?

DHx
- On any medication? Any doses of medication changed?
- Any allergies?

FHx
- Any conditions run in the family? Specifically, I'd like to ask about muscle conditions? Nervous system conditions? Something called an autoimmune condition?
- Has anyone in the family ever been affected by sensations similar to the ones you're describing to me now?

SHx –
- Smoking/ Alcohol/ Recreational drugs
- Home environment? Support?
- Occupation – impact on life and on occupation?

Summarise and Thank
- I'd just like to summarise back to you to make sure I haven't missed anything
- Is there anything you'd like to talk about that we haven't quite addressed?
Thank you for talking to me and I wish you all the best

Differential Diagnosis

	Diagnosis	Features In History	Features In Investigations	Management
PERIPHERAL	**Diabetic neuropathy**	Progressive loss of sensation in extremities, possible history of falls, difficulty with fine motor skills, history of poor diabetes control	Loss of sensation in glove and stocking distribution, reduced proprioception	Improve diabetes medication and education, monitor for other complications (diabetic ulcers, diabetic retinopathy, nephropathy), analgesia for neuropathic pain
	Carpal tunnel	Altered sensation lateral half of hand, worse at night, helped by shaking hand, progressive	Positive Tinnel's and Phalen's test, normal sensation at rest, no weakness	Steroid injection, carpal tunnel release
CENTRAL	**Multiple sclerosis**	Sensation loss, non-anatomical distribution, worse with heat (after hot bath). History of neurological symptoms separated in space and time	MRI brain and spine shows demyelinating lesions correlating to neurological symptoms.	Neurology input Immunosuppression
	Stroke / TIA	Sudden onset unilateral loss of sensation in anatomical distribution, perhaps associated with weakness. History of risk factors (IHD, AF, HTN, cholesterol, DM)	CT head shows ischaemia or bleed, high blood pressure, high cholesterol	Consider thrombolysis for ischaemic stroke within 4h of symptoms Risk factor control and anti-platelet therapy

Also consider: Cervical Spondylosis, Peripheral Nerve Palsies e.g. Erb's /Klumpke's if associated with weakness

Investigations

Examination	Full neurological examination
Bedside	Blood pressure, blood glucose, urine dip, Carpal tunnel: Tinnel's and Phalen's test
Bloods	FBC, U&E, bone profile, vitamin B12, folate, HbA1c, LFTs
Imaging	CT head, XR c-spine → MRI cervical spine
Special	Nerve conduction studies

Marking Criteria ALTERED SENSATION	Marks	
	Awarded	Available
Washes hands at the start of the station		1
Introduces themselves – Including First name, last name and role		1
Patient details confirmed: Full name, Age/ D.O.B.		1
Explains purpose of consultation		1
Open question about what brings the patient in today + Clarification of any ambiguity		1
Handedness – Briefly enquires about handedness		0
Site – Enquires about exact location of weakness		1
Onset (Timeline) – Asks questions to provide a clear understanding of onset and progression - Onset/ Circumstance - Sudden vs. gradual - Fluctuations - Progression - Past episodes		3
Character - Obtains a description of the sensation		1
Radiation - Asks about sensations in other regions of body		1
Associated symptoms ■ **Symptoms** elicited are relevant and clearly directed at either arriving at a diagnosis or excluding other plausible diagnoses - Numbness/ Pins & Needles; Weakness; Pain; Wasting; Twitching - Eyes; Sphincter control ■ **Systems** queried are relevant to the complaint and adequate questions are asked for each symptom - Neurological; Anxiety; Constitutional		6
Timing - This has been done		0
Exacerbation/ Relief - Clearly asks if the patient has noticed any relieving/ exacerbating factors, providing appropriate examples if prompted (Ex. Exercise/ rest; heating/ cooling; Anxiety)		1
Severity - Subjective quantitative assessment of severity of sensations		1
Explores **Ideas, Concerns and Expectations**		3
Elicits relevant **Past Medical History** - DM; High BP; High cholesterol; Nervous system disease; Spinal cord problems		2
Elicits relevant **Drug History** including **Allergies**		2
Elicits relevant **Family History**		2
Elicits relevant **Social History** – including Smoking/ alcohol/ recreational drugs; **H**ome environment and support; **O**ccupation and impact on life		2
Closes consultation appropriately allowing the patient to ask any questions		1
Presentation: structured, concise		2
Appropriate Differential Diagnosis ± Investigations ± Management Plan		3
Examiner mark – professionalism and rapport		5
Patient mark – professionalism and rapport		5

Consultation	Presentation	Global marks patient	Global marks examiner	Total
30	5	5	5	45

45F with numbness in feet

HPC	Patient with numbness in her feet. Does not know how long. Realised they were numb when she struck her foot on a door. Feels that she has reduced sensation in all 5 toes. Present in both feet. Has not noticed any change in sensation on shin or calf. Does not feel weak and not clumsy but feel as if she is walking on woods (on bare foot walking). Can sleep without any problem and has not noticed any distracting tingling in legs/feet. Has not noticed change in colour of skin or pain in limbs. Has not noticed cracks or ulcers in foot but has to use lots of cream to keep them moist as feel skin is dry in feet.
PMHx	T1DM, diagnosed age 7. Well controlled
DHx	NKDA, insulin
SHx	Lives with husband. Works as sales assistant. No alcohol or smoking history.
FHx	Nil relevant
ICE	"Doctor, I'm concerned that this has something to do with my diabetes. What steps can I take to protect my feet?"
Ix	HbA1c, FBC, glucose, LFT, B12, folate, USS Doppler of legs and feet, ABPI, nerve conduction tests
Dx	Diabetic neuropathy
Tx	Foot care, appropriate foot wear, podiatrist, good glycaemic and BP control. If symptoms of neuropathy are worse try pharmacotherapy (use pain protocol: amitriptyline, duloxetine, pregabalin)

30F with numbness and pain

HPC	Patient presenting with 1-year history of numbness and tingling sensation in limbs. Also complaining of diffuse pain all over the body, especially in response to pressure on skin. Says she has been feeling very tired and every day is a struggle. She is very exhausted and unable to carry out things she was able to do in the past. Reports insomnia. No obvious trauma, no chest pain/SOB/headache/dizziness. No bladder bowel problems but she feels she is getting more forgetful and can be distracted easily. No fever, headache, twitching or rash. No tinnitus. No ataxia. Patient denies any change in strength, but says she is less able to feel herself move which makes her less able to function day to day.
PMHx	Anxiety, depression
DHx	Fluoxetine, NKDA
FHx	Nil relevant
SHx	Lives alone, works as secretary. No alcohol or smoking.
ICE	"Doctor, I can't cope with this anymore. This is driving me insane. I'm in so much pain all the time. I need you to do something!"
Ix	FBC, U&E, LFT, Vitamin B and folate, CT brain.
Dx	Fibromyalgia.
Tx	Pain relief, counselling, amitriptyline, sometimes gabapentin or pregabalin can be used.

50F with hot flushes and increased sensitivity

HPC	Patient with 6-month history of hot flushes and overall increased sensitivity. Says she has been feeling more emotional and tired as well. Complaining of sweating and shivering. Sweating is worse at night and she feels that it is so bad that she has to wake up at night to change clothes. Episodes have sudden onset and no specific triggers. Also complaining of difficulty in falling asleep. She feels that she is unable to focus and forgetful at times. She feels that she has reduced sex drive and it is painful too. Denies any weight loss, cough, SOB, chest pain, bowel changes or lumps and bumps anywhere. No infective symptoms. Generally, fit and well.
PMHx	Nil relevant
DHx	Nil regular.
SHx	Ex-smoker, quit when first child was born 20 years ago. Social alcohol intake, 8 units over the weekend
ICE	"Doctor, its driving me mad that I have these hot flushes and then I'm suddenly freezing. It's throwing me off and ruining my days."
Ix	FBC, FSH, LH, oestradiol levels, lipids, glucose
Dx	Menopause.
Tx	Up to patient. Explain risks and benefits of HRT, non-pharmacological therapy e.g. evening primrose oil. Consider risk of heart disease.

CARDIO-RESPIRATORY HISTORIES

CHEST PAIN
"WOCC SOCRATES"

"WIPE" – Introduce yourself, whilst gaining consent
- Wash hands
- Introduce self – "Hello, my name is X and I am a medical student"
- Patient details – "Could I ask your full name and age?"
- Explain – "I have been asked to speak with you about what brings you in, would that be alright?"

Open
- I understand you've come in with some chest pain, can you tell me a little more about that?
- **C**larification
- **C**onsider pain relief – You seem to be in a lot of pain. Have you been offered pain relief?

Site – Where exactly is the pain?

Onset
- When did the pain start? Did anything happen around then?
- Did the pain come on suddenly or gradually?
- Does the pain come and go or is it continuous?
- Has the pain gotten progressively worse?
- Have you had this pain before?

Character – Can you describe the pain?
- **Crushing** (MI/ Angina), **Tearing** (Aortic dissection), **Sharp** (PE/ Tension pneumothorax/ Pericarditis/ Pneumonia/ MSK), **Burning** (GORD)

Radiation – Does the pain travel anywhere else?
- To arm/ neck or jaw (MI/ Angina)

Associated features
- Symptoms
  - ➤ **Sweating** – Have you been sweating due to the pain?
  - ➤ **Nausea** – Have you been nauseated due to the pain?
  - ➤ **Meals** – Is the pain related to meals at all? (Biliary colic? GORD?)
  - ➤ **Fever** – Have you felt unwell / hot and cold (infection – pneumonia, pericarditis, myocarditis)
- Systems
  - ➤ **Cardiovascular** – Any palpitations? Any LOC? Any SOB? Do you get breathless when lying flat? At night? How many pillows do you sleep with? Have you noticed swelling of your ankles or lower back?
  - ➤ **Respiratory** – Do you have any SOB? Any cough? ±blood? ±sputum? Any wheezing when you breathe?
  - ➤ **Musculoskeletal** – Does movement / taking a deep breath make it worse? Is the area tender?
  - ➤ **Constitutional** – Have you felt tired? Loss of appetite? Weight loss?

Timing – This has been done.

Exacerbating/ relieving
- Does anything make the pain better or worse?
  - ➤ Does **breathing in** make it worse? – pleuritic (PE / pneumonia)
  - ➤ Does **exercising/ excitement** make it worse – Angina
  - ➤ Does **sitting forwards** make it better / worse– pericarditis
  - ➤ Does **rest** relieve the pain? – Stable angina

Severity – How bad is the pain on a scale of 0 to 10? 0 being no pain and 10 being the worst pain imaginable.

ICE
- You've given me a lot of information, thank you. I'd like to hear a little about what you think could be going on. Do you have any idea?
- Is there anything that's particularly concerning you that you'd like to discuss?
- What did you hope I could help you with today? (resolution vs. reassurance)

PMHx
- Do you have any medical conditions / anything you take regular medications for?
- Ask a few specific questions to show that you're thinking about different causes
  - Ask about any past blood clots – PE?
- Specifically, I'd like to ask if you've ever been diagnosed with:
  - Heart problems? Angina? High BP? High cholesterol? Diabetes?

DHx
- On any medication? Any recent changes in medication or doses?
  - Specifically ask about the OCP
- Any allergies? What happens if you take it?

FHx
- Any conditions run in the family? Specifically, I'd like to ask about heart attacks? Blood clots? High cholesterol? High BP? Diabetes? Sudden death?
- Has anyone in the family ever been affected by chest pain similar to this?

SHx –
- Smoking/ Alcohol/ Recreational drugs (Especially COCAINE – coronary artery spasm)
- Home environment? Support?
- Occupation – impact on life and on occupation?

Summarise and Thank
- I'd just like to summarise back to you to make sure I haven't missed anything
- Is there anything you'd like to talk about that we haven't quite addressed?
- Thank you for talking to me and I wish you all the be

Top Tip!

Clubbing is a common exam favourite with examiners. Whilst around 40% of people with clubbing will have nothing wrong with them (idiopathic), the remaining will have serious pathology. Its worth your time learning the main causes of clubbing:

Respiratory: (ABCDEF)
- **A**bscess/ Asbestosis
- **B**ronchiectasis
- **C**ystic fibrosis
- **D**o NOT say COPD
- **E**mpyema
- **F**ibrosis

Cardiac:
Infective Endocarditis & Cyanotic heart disease

Gastrointestinal: (All C's)
Liver **C**irhosis, Ulcerative **C**olitis, Crohn's Disase, Hepatocellular **C**arcinoma

Differential Diagnosis

	Diagnosis	Features In History	Features In Investigations	Management
CARDIOVASCULAR	ACS	Central, heavy/dull, severe pain radiating to shoulder and jaw, associated with SOB, nausea, sweats, not relieved with rest or GTN. PMHx of angina. RF for cardiovascular disease (HTN, DM, cholesterol, obesity, FH, smoking)	ECG – ST segment and T wave changes or no ECG changes. Troponin may be raised (NSTEMI or STEMI) and should be done on admission and repeated 12h post symptom onset. May be normal in Unstable angina. Previous positive angiogram, MPS or cardiac MRI	300mg Aspirin, analgesia, anti-emetics Further management depending on whether PCI available and STEMI vs. NSTEMI
	Stable Angina	Dull central chest pain reproducible on exertion, relieved with rest and GTN, may radiate to shoulder. RF for cardiovascular disease as above.	No ECG changes, normal troponin. Inducible ischaemia in MPS or cardiac MRI. High HbA1c, cholesterol.	Risk factor management (statin, DM control, smoking cessation, weight loss, BP control) GTN spray PRN.
	Pericarditis	Central chest pain, sharp, pleuritic, better leaning forward, worse lying down, preceding viral infection, breathless, dizzy. Consider uraemic pericarditis in CKD.	Auscultate for pericardial rub (walking in snow) ECG: generalised saddle shaped T waves CXR: if pericardial effusion present – globular heart. Raised WCC, CRP Echo: may show effusion	NSAIDs regularly with gastric protection (PPI cover). Consider admission if haemodynamic compromise, septic or anticoagulated.
MUSCULOSKELETAL	Costochondritis	Sharp pleuritic chest pain, previous trauma possible, no radiation, no SOB / N&V / systemic illness. Well otherwise, no cardiac RFs	Tender on palpation of chest wall, lump may be palpable Nil findings on other investigations	NSAIDs and reassurance
	Trauma	History of blunt trauma or high impact injury	Rib Fractures on CXR. May co-exist with a pneumothorax	Resuscitate and transfer to Trauma/cardiac centre depending on severity

	Diagnosis	Features In History	Features In Investigations	Management
RESPIRATORY	**Pulmonary Embolism**	Pleuritic sharp chest pain, SOB, cough (maybe haemoptysis), RF for PE (immobilisation, surgery, COCP, pregnant, long journey), preceding swollen painful calf, previous / FH of PE	Reduced saturations, CXR may show wedge of reduced vascularisation, ECG: most common – sinus tachycardia, (rarely S1Q3T) Raised D-dimer Thrombus on CTPA or VQ mismatch in V/Q scan.	Anticoagulation (3 months for provoked, 6 months for unprovoked PE minimum), consider thrombophilia testing if recurrent. Thrombolysis if Haemodynamically compromised.
	Pneumothorax	Pleuritic chest pain, SOB with sudden onset, history of previous pneumothoraxes, tall thin stature or history of COPD with bullae / recent cardiac surgery. <u>Look for signs of haemodynamic compromise</u> – tachycardic, light headed, collapse	Reduced breath sounds on affected side, increased resonance to percussion, reduced expansion. CXR shows reduced vascular markings/ lung edge seen. BP may be low if tension pneumothorax.	If tension pneumothorax – immediate decompression with large bore cannula in 2nd intercostal space. If simple, drain if >2cm unless secondary to COPD
	Pneumonia	Pleuritic pain with SOB. History of fever and cough (frequently productive).	Consolidation on CXR, raised CRP and WCC on bloods.	Empirical Antibiotics, Sputum Culture, Paracetamol
GASTROINTESTINAL	**GORD**	Burning central chest pain, worse lying down and leaning forward, worse after meals, obesity, not Exertional, may radiate towards neck	Normal ECG, CXR may show hiatus hernia. Positive urea breath test if *H. Pylori*.	PPI and simple antacids. Weight loss. Consider *H. pylori* as cause and eradicate.

Investigations

Examination	Full cardiovascular and respiratory examination. Chest wall palpation.
Bedside	Blood pressure, blood glucose, oxygen saturations, ECG
Bloods	FBC, CRP, Troponin, D-dimer, U&E
Imaging	CXR
Special	Echocardiogram, CTPA or V/Q scan

Marking Criteria CHEST PAIN	Marks	
	Awarded	Available
Washed hands at the start of the station		1
Introduced themselves – Including First name, last name and role		1
Patient details confirmed: Full name, Age/ D.O.B.		1
Explained purpose of consultation		1
Open question about what brings the patient in today + Clarification of any ambiguity		1
Site – Enquires about exact location of chest pain		1
Onset (Timeline) – Asks questions to provide a clear understanding of onset and progression - Onset/ Circumstance - Sudden vs. gradual - Fluctuations - Progression - Past episodes		3
Character - Obtains an accurate description of the chest pain (Ex. Crushing, tearing, sharp, burning)		1
Radiation - Asks about the pain moving anywhere else (Ex. to arm/ jaw)		1
Associated symptoms ▪ **Symptoms** elicited are relevant and clearly directed at either arriving at a diagnosis or excluding other plausible diagnoses - Sweating - Nausea - Meals - Fever ▪ **Systems** queried are relevant to the complaint and adequate questions are asked for each symptom - Cardiovascular; Respiratory; Musculoskeletal; Constitutional		6
Timing - This has been done		0
Exacerbation/ Relief - Clearly asks if the patient has noticed any relieving/ exacerbating factors, providing appropriate examples if prompted (Ex. Breathing; sitting forwards; rest)		1
Severity - Subjective quantitative assessment of chest pain severity		1
Explores **Ideas, Concerns and Expectations**		3
Elicits relevant **Past Medical History** - Heart problems; angina; high cholesterol; DM; HTN		2
Elicits relevant **Drug History** including **Allergies**		2
Elicits relevant **Family History**		2
Elicits relevant **Social History** – including Smoking/ alcohol/ recreational drugs; Home environment and support; Occupation and impact on life		2
Closes consultation appropriately allowing the patient to ask any questions		1
Presentation: structured, concise		2
Appropriate Differential Diagnosis ± Investigations ± Management Plan		3
Examiner mark – professionalism and rapport		5
Patient mark – professionalism and rapport		5

Consultation	Presentation	Global marks patient	Global marks examiner	Total
— 30	— 5	— 5	— 5	— 45

67M, presenting with 2 hours of chest pain

HPC	Central, heavy pain, 9/10 severity, started suddenly whilst watching TV 2 hours ago, radiates to both shoulders and left jaw, associated with shortness of breath, has been feeling clammy, vomited x1. Not relieved with painkillers, not positional / pleuritic / related to eating. No fever / cough / recent travel / calf tenderness. No palpitations / orthopnoea / PND / peripheral oedema. "Spray under the tongue" helped a bit, but came back. Has had his pain before, but usually gets it walking up the hill to town. Last few days has been getting it briefly on and off whilst sitting at home. Normally relieved with GTN.
PMH	Femoral-popliteal bypass graft, appendicectomy, gall bladder.
DH	Aspirin, GTN, amlodipine, ramipril, furosemide, atorvastatin. NKDA.
FH	Father had MI at 58. Mother had stroke at 77.
SH	Retired, worked as builder. Lives with wife who is well. Smoker, 20/day for 45 years; 3 pints every night. Nil recreational drugs.
ICE	"I just want the pain to go away".
Dx	Myocardial Infarction
Ix	ECG, troponin
Mx	Analgesia, GTN, aspirin, ticagrelor, enoxaparin / angiogram depending on ECG, CCU admission.

38F, presenting with 6 hours of chest pain

HPC	Left sided chest pain, first started 6 hours ago, noticed it gradually and got worse, now 9/10 at worst, sharp, worse with taking a big breath, coughing up sputum (sometimes pink/red), slightly feverish, short of breath with minimal activity – started at the same time as the chest pain, bit dizzy. No radiation / trauma to chest / previous chest pain / relation to food / recent chest infection, PND, orthopnoea, oedema, chest wall tenderness. Travelled back from South Africa 2 weeks ago. Has noted her left calf has been a bit swollen and sore for 5 days ("been walking a lot recently").
PMH	Asthma, tonsillectomy, 2 x C-sections
DH	Salbutamol, seretide, combined contraceptive pill, vitamins. Allergic to penicillin – swelling of mouth and tongue.
FH	Mother- lung cancer. Father – diabetes, HTN, CABG at 55.
SH	Lives with husband, mother of 2 kids, works as receptionist. Non-smoker, social, 3 glasses of wine once a month.
ICE	"Scared I'm having a heart attack!"
Dx	Pulmonary Embolism
Ix	(Calculate Well's score) CXR, ECG, V/Q or CTPA.
Mx	O_2, anti-coagulation for 3 months at least (can calculate HAS-BLED for bleeding risk).

45M presents with 2 days of chest pain

HPC	2 days of central chest pain, achey all the time and sometimes sharp, worse lying flat, better leaning forward, getting more breathless over the 2 days – even at rest, has been feeling hot and cold for a few days, reduced appetite. No radiation, pleuritic chest pain, sweats, nausea, PND, trauma to chest, tenderness, cough, sputum.
PMH	Dislocated shoulder, torn anterior cruciate ligament
DH	Nil prescription meds. OTC: vitamins, fish oil. NKDA
SH	Gym instructor, lives with wife and son – son was ill with cough and cold recently. Smokes 3-4 cigarettes a day for 20 years, no alcohol, sometimes smokes marijuana
ICE	"Maybe I worked out too hard last week?"
Dx	Pericarditis
Ix	ECG, CXR, bloods incl. FBC, troponin and CRP, echo.
Mx	Oxygen if needed, cardiac monitor, anti-inflammatories, consider need for anti-viral/antibiotics

22 year old male presents with chest pain

HPC	Patient with acute onset left sided chest pain. Reports no trauma. Says he was sat at work and suddenly felt a stabbing pain in his chest. Says he feels short of breath and is struggling to breath. Patient does not report any palpitations, dizziness, nausea or vomiting. Pain is not radiating. Not sweating. Patient says he has never had this before.
PMH	Nil, investigated for Marfans syndrome in the past due to tall and skinny stature, no diagnosis made.
DH	Nil regular. PRN paracetamol. NKDA
FH	Adopted
SH	Student, physics. Social alcohol. Never smoked.
ICE	"I can't breathe doctor, I'm very worried"
Dx	Pneumothorax
Ix	CXR, ECG, U&E, LFT, FBC, cultures to rule out infection
Mx	Chest drain and monitor

45 year old female with central chest pain

HPC	Patient with recurring episodes of central crushing chest pain. Says the pain comes on after large meals and usually lasts for the entire day, progressively gets "less bad". Improved by drinking milk. Says pain is mainly limited to left, does not appear to be radiating. She feels short of breath and nauseous. No vomiting. No palpitations, no headache.
PMH	T2DM
DH	NKDA, Metformin, Aspirin, Atorvastatin
FH	Father diagnosed with gastric cancer age 50
SH	Drinks 25 units per week, 20 pack year history of smoking
ICE	"Doctor, I'm really worried I have a heart attack. I had a look on Google and the symptoms fit."
Dx	GORD
Ix	ECG, chest X-ray, FBC, U&E, LFT, troponin, endoscopy
Mx	Trial of PPI e.g. Omeprazole

55 year old male with chest pain

HPC	Patient presents with one week of intermittent chest pain. Associated with exercise. Chest pain is central and tight feeling. Not radiating, no nausea or vomiting. No sweating. Pain usually settles after a few moments of rest. Patient reports shortness of breath. Patient does not report any decrease in exercise tolerance over last months. Patient also reports tightness in his calves when walking for extended periods of time. Says it feels like the stitches.
PMH	T2DM, HTN
DHx	Insulin, Bisoprolol
FH	Father had MI age 50, mother diagnosed with T1DM in childhood
SH	Smoker. No alcohol, tee total now following alcohol dependency 5 years ago.
ICE	"Doctor, this chest pain is terrible. I'm really worried I'm having a heart attack like my dad."
Dx	Stable Angina
Ix	ECG, Echo, stress ECG, LFT, U&E, Troponin, CRP, Chest x-ray
Mx	GTN PRN, statin, aspirin, smoking cessation, ensure optimal BM control Consider other anti-anginals if no improevement e.g. ISMN and Ranolazine

PALPITATIONS
GENERAL FRAMEWORK

"WIPE" – Introduce yourself, whilst gaining consent
- Wash hands
- Introduce self – "Hello, my name is X and I am a medical student"
- Patient details – "Could I ask your full name and age?"
- Explain – "I have been asked to speak with you about what brings you in, would that be alright?"

Open
- Open – "I understand you've been feeling your heart racing recently. Could you tell me about that?"
- Clarify –

Timeline
1. When did you first notice this? Did anything happen then? (exercise/ anxiety…)
2. Did it come on suddenly or gradually?
3. Does it come and go or is it there all the time? What starts / stops it? (Manoeuvres/ drugs…)
4. Has it been getting worse?
5. Have you ever had anything like this before?

Symptoms
- Palpitations (Think of a timeline: pre, during, after)
    - **Precipitants** – If you have not yet elicited this information ask specifically what triggers these palpitations – anxiety/ exercise/ coffee/ standing up?
    - **Rhythm** – Are these palpitations regular or irregular? Can you tap them out for me?
    - **Sweat** – Do you feel sweaty when these palpitations come on?
    - **Nausea** – Do you feel nauseous when these palpitations come on?
    - **Faintness** – Do you feel light-headed when these palpitations come on? Have you ever fallen or blacked out?
    - **Duration** – How long do they last when they do come on?
    - **Termination** – Do they stop by alone or do you have to do something to stop them?
    - How do you feel after they stop?
- Others
    - **Thyroid** – Have you been especially intolerant of heat? Have you lost any weight? How have your bowels been? Have you noticed a tremor? Have you felt anxious? More personal question. How have your periods been?

Systems
- **Cardiovascular** – Do you get any chest pain? Have you lost consciousness? Do you feel SOB? Do you ever get breathless lying down or at night? How many pillows do you sleep with? Have you noticed swelling in your ankles or lower back?
- **Anxiety** – Are you an anxious person or have you been anxious recently? Do you think this could be related?
- **Constitutional** – any weight loss? Fevers? Loss of appetite?

ICE
- You've given me a lot of information, thank you. I'd like to hear a little about what you think could be going on. Do you have any idea?
- Is there anything that's particularly concerning you that you'd like to discuss?
- What exactly are you looking for today, resolution or reassurance?

PMHx
- Do you have any medical conditions?
- Ask a few specific questions to show that you're thinking about different causes
- Specifically, I'd like to ask if you've ever been diagnosed with:
  - ➢ Heart problems? (E.g. HF, Arrhythmia) Thyroid problems? Anxiety/ Panic attacks? Asthma?

DHx
- On any medication? Any doses of medication changed?
  - ➢ Specifically ask: Any inhalers? Lots of coffee or tea?
- Any allergies?

FHx
- Any conditions run in the family? Specifically, I'd like to ask about heart problems? Thyroid disease? Sudden death?
- Has anyone in the family ever had palpitations similar to the ones you're experiencing now?

SHx –
- Smoking/ Alcohol/ Recreational drugs
- Home environment? Support?
- Occupation – impact on life and on occupation?

Summarise and Thank
- I'd just like to summarise back to you to make sure I haven't missed anything
- Is there anything you'd like to talk about that we haven't quite addressed?
- Thank you for talking to me and I wish you all the best

Investigations

Examination	Cardiovascular examination, thyroid examination
Bedside	Blood pressure, ECG, blood glucose, urine dip
Bloods	FBC, CRP, U&E, TFTs, troponin, alcohol levels
Imaging	CXR, echocardiogram
Special	24 hour Holter monitor, urine catecholamines, anxiety screen

Differential Diagnosis

	Diagnosis	Features In History	Features In Investigations	Management
CARDIAC	SVT	Random onset palpitations, fast regular, some shortness of breath, may be terminated with Valsalva manoeuvres. NO cardiac risk factors, often young.	Normal ECG at rest, sinus tachycardia with palpitations	Valsalva manoeuvres, carotid massage, cold water face wash. "Pill in pocket" beta blocker.
	Atrial fibrillation	Random onset (may be after alcohol or caffeine), fast irregular heartbeat, associated with light-headedness, chest pain, SOB. May have history of stroke/ TIA, CCF (PND, oedema, orthopnoea), MI, murmur (ass. With MR)	Irregularly irregular pulse, ECG: no P waves, irregularly irregular. Signs of CCF	Calculate CHA2DS2-VASc for anticoagulation for stroke risk (also calculate HASBLED)
HORMONAL	Hyperthyroidism	Often young. Palpitations (may be regular or irregular), sweats, weight loss, diarrhoea, anxiety, increased appetite, irregular periods, heat intolerance	Hand tremor, tachycardia, diaphoretic. ECG: sinus tachycardia or AF. TFTs: raised T4 suppressed TSH (in primary hyperthyroidism)	Commonly "Block and replace" with carbimazole and thyroxine in primary. Look for goitre, thyroid cancer and pituitary mass for secondary.
OTHER	Anxiety	Chest discomfort, fast heartbeat, anxious, may have depression / stressors in life. Loss of appetite and energy if also depressed.	Normal ECG and bloods.	CBT, psychotherapy, propranolol.
Also consider: Heart block, caffeine and phaeochromocytoma				

Marking Criteria PALPITATIONS	Marks	
	Awarded	Available
Washes hands at the start of the station		1
Introduces themselves – Including First name, last name and role		1
Patient details confirmed: Full name, Age/ D.O.B.		1
Explains purpose of consultation		1
Open question about what brings the patient in today + Clarification of any ambiguity		1
Timeline allows a clear understanding of onset and progression - Onset/ Circumstance - Sudden vs. gradual - Fluctuations - Progression - Past episodes		3
Symptoms elicited are relevant and clearly directed at either arriving at a diagnosis or excluding other plausible diagnoses o Precipitants o Rhythm o Sweating o Nausea o Faintness o Duration o Termination o Thyroid specific		5
Systems queried are relevant to the complaint and adequate questions are asked for each symptom - Cardiovascular; Anxiety; Constitutional		5
Explores **Ideas, Concerns and Expectations**		3
Elicits relevant **Past Medical History** - Heart problems; Thyroid problems; Anxiety/ Panic attacks; Asthma		2
Elicits relevant **Drug History** including **Allergies**		2
Elicits relevant **Family History**		2
Elicits relevant **Social History** – including Smoking/ alcohol/ recreational drugs; **Home** environment and support; **Occupation** and impact on life		2
Closes consultation appropriately allowing the patient to ask any questions		1
Presentation: structured, concise		2
Appropriate Differential Diagnosis ± Investigations ± Management Plan		3
Examiner mark – professionalism and rapport		5
Patient mark – professionalism and rapport		5

Consultation	Presentation	Global marks patient	Global marks examiner	Total
30	5	5	5	45

71M presents with "a funny feeling in his chest"

HPC	Had a funny feeling in his chest for the last 1 ½ days, heart racing, funny rhythm (can't tap out, irregular), fast, comes and goes, makes him feel short of breath and slightly light headed, never had it before, has noted ankle swelling today, slight tightness in the chest with it. Diarrhoea and fever for 4 days associated with nausea, abdominal pain, reduced appetite, "under the weather" and tired for around a week. No cough / weight loss / stress / anxiety / new medications / change in medications / caffeine / alcohol
PMH	CABG when 68 years old, cholecystectomy, HTN, T2DM, hypercholesterolaemia, COPD
DH	Aspirin, atorvastatin, amlodipine, losartan, salbutamol, symbicort, metformin. Allergic: ramipril cough.
FH	Father died of "bleed in the brain", mother lived till 101 years old
SH	Lives with wife who had D&V last week, normally independent ADLs but gets weekly cleaner and children help with shopping. Ex-smoker, 20/day for 50 years. No alcohol or drugs.
ICE	"Has my bypass stopped working, doctor?"
Dx	Atrial fibrillation (secondary to gastroenteritis).
Ix	ECG (no p-waves, new MI?), observations (haemodynamically stable?), CXR (?pulmonary oedema). Calculate CHA_2DS_2-VASc.
Mx	Treat underlying cause, consider need for anti-coagulation.

27F with a racing heart

HPC	Heart racing started suddenly 3 hours ago, has had several times in last 6 months but usually stop by themselves in 3-5 minutes, making her feel anxious, some shortness of breath and hyperventilating, feels dizzy with it, feels very fast but regular, was just walking to work when it started but previous episodes also at rest – random on and offset, nothing making it worse or better. Drinks 5 cups of coffee a day. No LOC / previous heart conditions / cough / weight loss / diarrhoea / recent infection / oedema / PND / orthopnoea / new medications / drug use / chest pain
PMH	Nil
DH	Combined contraceptive pill, vitamins
FH	Mother has atrial fibrillation
SH	Lives with a friend, works in a bank. Smoker, 5-7 a day for 5 years. One bottle of wine at weekends. Occasional drug use – marijuana, cocaine, none in the last fortnight.
ICE	"Do I need to have blood thinning like my mother does for her abnormal heart beat?"
Dx	Paroxysmal SVT.
Ix	ECG, Bloods incl. FBC (?anaemia), TFT (?hyperthyroid) , U&E (?electrolyte abnormality).
Mx	Cardioversion if haemodynamic compromise. Vagal manoeuvres, adenosine / CCBs / beta-blockers.

39F presents with fast heart beat

HPC	Has noticed she always seems to have a fast heart beat (around 100 beats per minute), sometimes feels tight chested with it but occasionally very aware of heart beat, makes her feel anxious and short of breath. Heartbeat is regular. Noticed she appears to feel hotter than her co-workers, losing weight but not trying to, increased appetite, opening bowels more often, irregular periods (were regular 1 year ago), finding it hard to work as her hands shake, feels anxious more ("work is very stressful"). Husband says her eyes look bigger "like I'm scared or surprised all the time" No LOC / orthopnoea / PND / oedema / chest pain / cough
PMH	Vitiligo, IBS
DH	Steroid cream. NKDA
FH	Mother had vitiligo and coeliac. Sister has T1DM.
SH	Lives with husband, works as a hospital nurse. Smokes 5/day, 10 years. Drinks socially - few glasses of wine at weekends
ICE	"I've been losing a lot of weight… Have I got cancer?"
Dx	Hyperthyroidism (likely Grave's).
Ix	Thyroid examination, ECG, CXR, TFTs.
Mx	Beta blocker, endocrinology referral

SHORTNESS OF BREATH
GENERAL FRAMEWORK

"WIPE" – Introduce yourself, whilst gaining consent
- Wash hands
- Introduce self – "Hello, my name is X and I am a medical student"
- Patient details – "Could I ask your full name and age?"
- Explain – "I have been asked to speak with you about what brings you in, would that be alright?"

Open
- Open – I understand you've been feeling breathless recently. Could you tell me about that?
- Clarify

Timeline
1. When did you start feeling SOB? What were you doing / what happened then?
2. Did you suddenly feel SOB or did it come on gradually?
3. Does it come and go or are you breathless all the time? (Seasonal variation?)
4. Is it getting worse?
5. Have you ever been SOB like this before?

Symptoms
- Breathlessness
  - ➤ **Severity?** – How bad is the breathlessness? How much does it affect your day-to-day life? Try to quantify according to **MRC Scale** (see below)
  - ➤ **When?** – When do you become breathless? Does it change with seasons/ over the course of the day (E.g. asthma)?
  - ➤ **Relieving/ Exacerbating?** – Does anything relieve the breathlessness? Have you tried any inhalers?
- Risk – **"TIE TAP"**
  - ➤ **Travel** – Have you been on any long-haul flights recently? (PE) Have you travelled anywhere outside of the UK recently? (TB/ Infection)
  - ➤ **Illness** – Have you been ill recently? (Pneumonia)
  - ➤ **Exposure** – Is there any chance you've been exposed to asbestos/ farming/ organic dusts/ birds? (Can ask here or with SHx) (Asbestosis, cancer, hypersensitivity pneumonitis)
  - ➤ **Trauma** – Have you had any recent fractures? (PE)
  - ➤ **Allergens** – Have you been exposed to dust / pollen / pets? (Asthma)?
  - ➤ **Pregnancy** – Is there any change you could be pregnant? (PE)

Systems
- **Cardiovascular** – Do you get any chest pain? Have you lost consciousness? Do you feel SOB? Do you ever get breathless lying down or at night? How many pillows do you sleep with? Have you noticed swelling in your ankles or lower back?
- **Respiratory** – Do you get any chest pain? Wheeze? Cough? ±Blood ±Sputum
- **Anxiety** – Are you an anxious person? Do you think it could be related?
- **Constitutional** – How has your appetite been? Have you noticed a change in weight? Fevers? Night-sweats? Hoarseness/ dysphagia/ wheezing/ stridor?

ICE
- You've given me a lot of information, thank you. I'd like to hear a little about what you think could be going on. Do you have any idea?
- Is there anything that's particularly concerning you that you'd like to discuss?
- What exactly are you looking for today, resolution or reassurance?

PMHx
- Do you have any medical conditions?
- Ask a few specific questions to show that you're thinking about different causes
- Specifically, I'd like to ask if you've ever been diagnosed with:
    - Heart disease? Respiratory infections? Asthma/ eczema/ hay-fever? A blood clot? COPD? Cancer? Tuberculosis?

DHx
- On any medication? Any doses of medication changed?
    - Specifically ask: OCP? Inhalers?
- Any allergies?

FHx
- Any conditions run in the family? Specifically, I'd like to ask about asthma/ eczema/ hay-fever (atopy)? Tuberculosis? Heart problems?
- Is anyone else in the family experiencing the same symptoms as you at the moment? (Infectious cause) And what about in the past? (FHx)

SHx –
- SMOKING (COPD/ Malignancy)/ Alcohol/ Recreational drugs
- Home environment? Support?
- OCCUPATION (ASBESTOS?/ FARMING?)– impact on life and on occupation?

Summarise and Thank
- I'd just like to summarise back to you to make sure I haven't missed anything
- Is there anything you'd like to talk about that we haven't quite addressed?
- Thank you for talking to me and I wish you all the best

Medical Research Council (MRC) Dyspnoea Scale

Grade	Impact
0	Not troubled by breathlessness except during strenuous exercise
1	Breathless when hurrying on the level or walking up a slight hill
2	Walks slower than most OR stops for breath when walking at own pace at level
3	Stops for breath after walking 100m OR after a few minutes on the level
4	Too breathless to leave the house OR breathless or dressing/ undressing

Differential Diagnosis

	Diagnosis	Features In History	Features In Investigations	Management
ACUTE	**Pneumothorax**	Sudden onset pleuritic chest pain, history of previous pneumothoraxes, tall thin stature or history of COPD with bullae / recent cardiac surgery. <u>Look for signs of haemodynamic compromise</u> – tachycardia, light headedness, collapse	<u>Examination</u>: Reduced breath sounds on affected side, increased resonance to percussion, reduced expansion. CXR shows reduced vascular markings/ lung edge seen. BP may be low if tension pneumothorax.	If tension pneumothorax – immediate decompression with large bore cannula in 2nd intercostal space. If simple, drain if >2cm unless secondary to COPD
	Acute Asthma / COPD	Acute onset SOB with exercise / pollen / pets with wheeze. History of asthma / COPD. Preceding viral infection, productive cough. Worse at night. Helped by Salbutamol inhalers.	<u>Examination</u>: reduced expansion, bilateral wheeze (silent chest is a bad sign), tachypnoea, reduced saturations. Reduced peak flow. CXR: may see focus of infection. Hyper inflated lungs in chronic asthma/ COPD Obstructive pattern on spirometry (asthma has reversibility with bronchodilators)	Oxygen if reduced saturations, Salbutamol and ipratropium nebuliser / inhaler, antibiotics if infective cause. Stretch inhalers as tolerated. Education on control and up-titrate preventative medication.
	Anaphylaxis	Acute onset shortness of breath after new food / medication, chest tightness, sweats, red rash, itchy, abdominal pain, nausea and vomiting, difficulty breathing, faint.	<u>Examination</u>: Stridor, tachypnoea, urticarial rash, tongue / lip swelling, wheeze on auscultation of chest. Bloods may show raised tryptase.	Immediate IM adrenaline 0.5ml 1:1000, oxygen, IV fluids, steroids, anti-histamines. Monitor for rebound anaphylaxis.
	Pulmonary Embolism	Pleuritic sharp chest pain, SOB, cough (maybe haemoptysis), RF for PE (immobilisation, surgery, COCP, pregnant, long journey), preceding swollen painful calf, previous / FH of PE	Examination- Reduced saturations, CXR may show wedge of reduced vascularisation, ECG: most common – sinus tachycardia, (rarely S1Q3T). Raised D-dimer. Thrombus on CTPA or VQ mismatch in V/Q scan. Tachypnoea	Anticoagulation (3 months for provoked, 6 months for unprovoked PE minimum), consider thrombophilia testing if recurrent. Thrombolysis if Haemodynamically compromised.
	For Acute SOB also consider: Foreign body and Anxiety			

	Diagnosis	Features In History	Features In Investigations	Management
CHRONIC	**Pulmonary oedema / congestive cardiac failure**	Progressive shortness of breath, orthopnoea, PND, cough of frothy pink sputum, no fever, ankle oedema, history of cardiac disease, cardiac risk factors (HTN, DM, FHx, smoking, lipids, obesity)	Reduced saturation, tachypnoea, bilateral crackles on examination / reduced air entry and dullness to percussion if effusion present, pitting oedema, S3 heart sound of volume overload. CXR: fluid overload Bloods: raised BNP Echo: reduced ejection fraction	Offload fluid with diuretics, monitor U&Es, disease modifying medications of heart failure and symptomatic relief (ACEi, spironolactone, beta blocker)
	Lung Fibrosis	Long history of progressive shortness of breath. No cough, no wheeze, no change with inhalers, no triggers. History of working in coal mining / bakery / farm or medications known to cause fibrosis	Fine end inspiratory crepitations (apical vs. basal for causes) High resolution CT chest – ground glass shadowing and honeycombing Restrictive picture on spirometry	Immunosuppression and regular follow up. Cease triggering factors.
	Lung cancer	Progressive history of shortness of breath, haemoptysis, chronic cough. B-symptoms: fevers, lethargy, appetite loss, weight loss, anorexia, sweats. History of smoking, FHx cancer.	May hear monophonic wheeze in bronchial cancer. Mass on CXR. CT chest – mass and lymphadenopathy.	MDT approach to consider resection vs. chemo/radiotherapy or combination. Smoking cessation.
	Pneumonia	Pleuritic pain with SOB. History of fever and cough (frequently productive).	Consolidation on CXR, raised CRP and WCC on bloods.	Empirical Antibiotics, Sputum Culture, Paracetamol
	For Chronic SOB also consider: Pleural effusion (secondary to Heart Failure, Cancer) and Anaemia			

Investigations

Examination	Respiratory and cardiac examination, ?full sentences
Bedside	Oxygen saturations, peak flow, ECG
Bloods	FBC, CRP, U&E, BNP, D-dimer, Arterial Blood Gas, Troponin
Imaging	CXR, CT chest, CTPA or V/Q scan
Special	Spirometry with reversibility

Marking Criteria SOB	Marks	
	Awarded	Available
Washes hands at the start of the station		1
Introduces themselves – Including First name, last name and role		1
Patient details confirmed: Full name, Age/ D.O.B.		1
Explains purpose of consultation		1
Open question about what brings the patient in today + Clarification of any ambiguity		1
Timeline allows a clear understanding of onset and progression - Onset/ Circumstance - Sudden vs. gradual - Fluctuations - Progression - Past episodes		3
Symptoms elicited are relevant and clearly directed at either arriving at a diagnosis or excluding other plausible diagnoses - Breathlessness o Severity o Timing o Relieving/ Exacerbating - Risk – "TIE TAP" o Travel o Illness o Exposure o Trauma o Allergens o Pregnancy		5
Systems queried are relevant to the complaint and adequate questions are asked for each symptom - Cardiovascular; Respiratory; Anxiety; Constitutional		5
Explores **Ideas, Concerns and Expectations**		3
Elicits relevant **Past Medical History** - Heart problems; Respiratory infections; asthma/ eczema/hay-fever; Blood clot; COPD; Cancer; TB		2
Elicits relevant **Drug History** including **Allergies**		2
Elicits relevant **Family History**		2
Elicits relevant **Social History** – including Smoking/ alcohol/ recreational drugs; **H**ome environment and support; **O**ccupation and impact on life		2
Closes consultation appropriately allowing the patient to ask any questions		1
Presentation: structured, concise		2
Appropriate Differential Diagnosis ± Investigations ± Management Plan		3
Examiner mark – professionalism and rapport		5
Patient mark – professionalism and rapport		5

Consultation	Presentation	Global marks patient	Global marks examiner	Total
30	5	5	5	45

21F presents with shortness of breath

HPC	Sudden onset shortness of breath 2 hours ago whilst at a friend's house, nothing is making it worse, her "blue inhaler" helped a bit, feels tight in the chest, wheezy, finding it hard to talk for long periods, not able to walk quickly Been getting a cough at night and mornings – non-productive, gets a bit wheezy when exercising but resolves by itself, gets wheezy when she has colds/coughs. No chest pain / productive cough / recent travel / PND / orthopnoea / ankle swelling / chest wall tenderness / pleuritic pain / new foods just before / rash / tongue swelling
PMH	Eczema, "viral wheeze" as a child,
DH	Creams for eczema, combined contraceptive pill. Allergic: penicillin – rash.
FH	Brother has eczema and hay-fever, mother has eczema, father has COPD
SH	Lives with flatmates, university student, smokes 4-5/day for 6 months, has 15-20 drinks socially a week, social marijuana use, nil other drugs.
ICE	"Have I got a collapsed lung like my mate had?"
Dx	Acute asthma
Ix	Peak flow, CXR.
Mx	Oxygen if needed, salbutamol (inhaler/nebulised), prednisolone

68F presents with worsening shortness of breath

HPC	Getting more breathless over the last two weeks, feeling tired all the time, worse on exertion, legs have been getting more swollen too, breathless lying flat (needing 3 pillows) and waking up at night gasping for air (3-4 times in last week). Has cough – productive – clear and frothy. No fever / recent travel / chest pain / wheeze / pleuritic pain / palpitations Recently stopped "water tablets" because it was affecting her kidneys.
PMH	HTN, hypercholesterolaemia, a heart valve problem, AF, COPD
DH	Amlodipine, warfarin, atorvastatin, aspirin, symbicort, salbutamol. Allergic: penicillin, codeine.
FH	Father and mother had blood pressure and heart troubles.
SH	Lives with husband who has dementia. Used to work in bakery. Smoker – 15/day for 50 years, nil alcohol.
ICE	"I can't look after my husband if I'm like this, what am I going to do?"
Dx	Pulmonary oedema (secondary to LV dysfunction).
Ix	CXR, bloods incl. BNP and U&Es.
Mx	Diuretics, fluid restriction, monitor U&Es

58M presents with shortness of breath

HPC	Sudden onset shortness of breath whilst at work, can't take a full breath, chest pain on the right side – worse when taking a deep breath, radiates to right shoulder, sharp/stabbing, pain started with SOB. No previous episodes / cough / wheeze / tongue swelling / rash / new food or meds / fevers / long journeys / calf swelling and tenderness
PMH	COPD, eczema
DH	Salbutamol, seretide.
FH	Nil
SH	Lives with wife, works as accountant. Smoker 30/day for 40 years, no alcohol or drugs.
ICE	"Is it my heart?"
Dx	Pneumothorax (secondary to COPD).
Ix	CXR, oxygen saturations
Mx	Drain or not depends on size of pneumothorax, conservative management of symptoms

COUGH
GENERAL FRAMEWORK

<u>**"WIPE"**</u> – Introduce yourself, whilst gaining consent
- Wash hands
- Introduce self – "Hello, my name is X and I am a medical student"
- Patient details – "Could I ask your full name and age?"
- Explain – "I have been asked to speak with you about what brings you in, would that be alright?"

<u>**Open**</u>
- Open – I understand you've come in with a cough. Can you tell me more about that?
- Clarify

<u>**Timeline**</u>
1. When did the cough start? Did anything happen/ were you doing anything then?
2. Did the cough come on suddenly or gradually?
3. Does the cough come and go or is it always there?
4. Has the cough been getting worse?
5. Have you ever had a cough like this before?

<u>**Symptoms**</u>
- **Cough**
  - ➢ **How bad?** – How bad is the cough? How much does it affect your day-to-day life?
  - ➢ **When?** – When does the cough come on? Does it change with seasons/ over the course of the day (E.g. asthma)?
  - ➢ **Relieving/ Exacerbating?** – Does anything relieve the cough? Have you tried any inhalers?
  - ➢ **Sputum** – Do you cough up any sputum? How much? How often? What does it look like?
    - ➢ Purulent green/ yellow sputum = bacterial
    - ➢ Rusty sputum = pneumonia
    - ➢ Frothy white sputum with blood = pulmonary oedema
  - ➢ **Blood** – Have you coughed up any blood? Is it red of dark? How much (splatters/ spoonfuls/ cupfuls)?
- Risk – **"TIE TAP"**
  - ➢ **Travel** – Have you been on any long-haul flights recently? (PE) Have you travelled anywhere outside of the UK recently? (TB/ Infection)
  - ➢ **Illness** – Have you been ill recently? Runny nose vs. generalised malaise (Flu vs. pneumonia).
  - ➢ **Exposure** – Is there any chance you've been exposed to asbestos/ farming/ organic dusts/ birds? (Can ask here or with SHx) (Asbestosis, cancer, hypersensitivity pneumonitis)
  - ➢ **Trauma** – Have you had any recent fractures? (PE)
  - ➢ **Allergens** – Have you been exposed to dust? Pets? (Asthma)
  - ➢ **Pregnancy** – Is there any change you could be pregnant? (PE)

<u>**Systems**</u>
- **Cardiovascular** – Do you get any chest pain? Have you lost consciousness? Do you feel SOB? Do you ever get breathless lying down or at night? How many pillows do you sleep with? Have you noticed swelling in your ankles or lower back?
- **Respiratory** – Do you get any chest pain? SOB? Wheeze?
- **Constitutional** – How has your appetite been? Have you noticed a change in weight? Fevers? Night-sweats? Hoarseness/ dysphagia/ wheezing/ stridor?

<u>**ICE**</u>
- You've given me a lot of information, thank you. I'd like to hear a little about what you think could be going on. Do you have any idea?
- Is there anything that's particularly concerning you that you'd like to discuss?
- What exactly are you looking for today, resolution or reassurance?

PMHx
- Do you have any medical conditions?
- Ask a few specific questions to show that you're thinking about different causes
- Specifically, I'd like to ask if you've ever been diagnosed with:
  - ➢ Heart disease? Respiratory infections? Asthma/ eczema/ hay-fever? A blood clot? COPD? Cancer? Tuberculosis?

DHx
- On any medication? Any doses of medication changed?
  - ➢ Specifically ask: OCP? Inhalers? BP medication (ACE-Inhibitors)?
- Any allergies?

FHx
- Any conditions run in the family? Specifically, I'd like to ask about asthma/ eczema/ hay-fever (atopy)? Tuberculosis? Heart problems? Lung problems? At what age? (Cystic Fibrosis/ alpha1-antitrypsin deficiency)
- Is anyone else in the family experiencing the same symptoms as you at the moment? (Infectious cause) And what about in the past? (FHx)

SHx –
- SMOKING (COPD/ Malignancy)/ Alcohol/ Recreational drugs
- Home environment? Support?
- OCCUPATION (ASBESTOS?/ FARMING?)– impact on life and on occupation?

Summarise and Thank
- I'd just like to summarise back to you to make sure I haven't missed anything
- Is there anything you'd like to talk about that we haven't quite addressed?
- Thank you for talking to me and I wish you all the best

Investigations

Examination	Respiratory and cardiac examination, ?full sentences
Bedside	Oxygen saturations, peak flow, temperature, blood pressure and pulse (?compromise)
Bloods	FBC, CRP, U&E, BNP. Consider alpha-1-antitrypsin if liver disease alluded to
Imaging	CXR, CT chest, CTPA or V/Q scan
Special	Spirometry with reversibility, sputum MC&S

Differential Diagnosis

	Diagnosis	Features In History	Features In Investigations	Management
SHORT TERM	**Pneumonia**	Productive cough, purulent sputum, SOB, fevers, appetite loss, myalgia, recent travel / ill contacts. May have pleuritic chest pain. Ask about confusion.	Tachypnoea. Coarse crackles and dullness to percussion in one area. Consolidation on CXR. Raised WCC and CRP on bloods. Bacterial growth from sputum.	Calculate CURB-65 for admission if high score. Antibiotics, oxygen if needed, IV fluids if dehydrated.
	Asthma / COPD	Cough, especially nocturnal, morning and exercise-associated, with wheeze and shortness of breath. Helped by Salbutamol inhalers. Asthma – triggered by exercise, pollen, pets. Associated with hay fever, eczema. COPD – history of smoking (usually 20+ pack years), chest infections in the winter, "smokers cough"	Examination: reduced expansion, bilateral wheeze, tachypnoea, reduced saturations. Reduced peak flow. CXR: may see focus of infection. Hyper inflated lungs in COPD. Obstructive pattern on spirometry (asthma has reversibility with bronchodilators)	Education on control and optimisation of preventative medication (see BTS guidelines) and Salbutamol reliever inhaler.
LONG TERM	**Drugs**	Dry cough, non-productive, no fever, not systemically unwell, no SOB or chest pain. Recently started ACEi	NO findings on examination, bloods or CXR	Stop ACEi and start alternative e.g. ARB
	Tuberculosis	Ongoing productive cough, weight loss, fevers, appetite loss, night sweats. Travel to endemic TB region in last year, or previous TB, no BCG vaccine.	CXR: apical consolidation. Bloods: raised WCC, CRP, quantiFERON +ve. Early morning sputum positive for acid fast bacilli.	Commence anti-TB treatment (RIPE for 2 months then RI for 4 months). Contact precautions in hospital.
	Lung Cancer	Chronic history of cough, haemoptysis, progressive shortness of breath. B-symptoms: fevers, lethargy, appetite loss, weight loss, sweats. History of smoking, FHx cancer.	May hear monophonic wheeze in bronchial cancer. Mass on CXR. CT chest – mass and lymphadenopathy.	MDT approach to consider resection vs. chemo/radiotherapy. Smoking cessation.
	EAA / fibrosis	Long history of progressive shortness of breath. No cough, no wheeze, no change with inhalers, no triggers. History of working in coal mining / bakery / farm or medications known to cause fibrosis (methotrexate, amiodarone, bleomycin etc.)	High resolution CT chest – ground glass shadowing and honeycombing Restrictive picture on spirometry	Immunosuppression and regular follow up. Cease triggering factors.
	Cystic Fibrosis	Chronic productive cough of white thick sputum, sometimes turning purulent with fevers and systemic upset.	Small for age, clubbed fingers, evidence of respiratory distress, cyanosis.	Referral to specialist MDT, sputum culture & empirical antibiotics

Marking Criteria Cough	Marks	
	Awarded	Available
Washes hands at the start of the station		1
Introduces themselves – Including First name, last name and role		1
Patient details confirmed: Full name, Age/ D.O.B.		1
Explains purpose of consultation		1
Open question about what brings the patient in today + Clarification of any ambiguity		1
Timeline allows a clear understanding of onset and progression - Onset/ Circumstance - Sudden vs. gradual - Fluctuations - Progression - Past episodes		3

Symptoms elicited are relevant and clearly directed at either arriving at a diagnosis or excluding other plausible diagnoses
- Cough
  o Severity
  o Timing
  o Relieving/ Exacerbating
  o Sputum
  o Blood
- Risk
  o Travel
  o Illness
  o Exposure
  o Trauma
  o Allergens
  o Pregnancy
		5

Systems queried are relevant to the complaint and adequate questions are asked for each symptom - Cardiovascular; Respiratory; Constitutional		5
Explores **Ideas, Concerns and Expectations**		3
Elicits relevant **Past Medical History** - Heart problems; Respiratory infections; asthma/ eczema/hay-fever; Blood clot; COPD; Cancer; TB		2
Elicits relevant **Drug History** including **Allergies**		2
Elicits relevant **Family History**		2
Elicits relevant **Social History** – including Smoking/ alcohol/ recreational drugs; **H**ome environment and support; **O**ccupation and impact on life		2
Closes consultation appropriately allowing the patient to ask any questions		1
Presentation: structured, concise		2
Appropriate Differential Diagnosis ± Investigations ± Management Plan		3
Examiner mark – professionalism and rapport		5
Patient mark – professionalism and rapport		5

Consultation	Presentation	Global marks patient	Global marks examiner	Total
30	5	5	5	45

35F presents with cough

HPC	Cough for the last 5 days, worsening, associated with fevers, tiredness, reduced appetite, muscle aches. It's disturbing sleep. Productive of sputum – brown/rust coloured, thick, no blood. Shortness of breath on exertion. Chest pain when coughing. Travelled to Spain last week, stayed at hotel near beach. No long journeys / wheeze / pleuritic pain / stridor / ankle swelling / orthopnoea / PND
PMH	Coeliac disease, hay fever.
DH	Combined contraceptive pill. NKDA
FH	Brother – asthma. Mother – arthritis.
SH	Works in office, lives with husband and children – all well. Ex-smoker, 5/day for 10 years. Social drinker - glass of wine at weekends.
ICE	"Is it TB?"
Dx	Pneumonia
Ix	CXR, bloods incl. FBC, CRP, sputum sample, calculate CURB-65
Mx	Oxygen if needed, antibiotics

49M presents with chronic cough

HPC	Cough ongoing for over a month. Started gradually, cough worsening – productive of light green sputum, increasing shortness of breath. Getting fevers most days. Not better despite antibiotics and steroids from the GP. Lethargy worsening over last few months, lost his appetite and lost 5kg in last 1 month, getting drenching night sweats occasionally every night for 2 weeks. Travelled home to India 2 months ago – stayed with family and friends. No wheeze / chest pain / PND / orthopnoea / oedema / new medications / pleuritic pain / calf swelling or tenderness
PMH	Asthma, T2DM, bad pneumonia as a child
DH	Metformin, salbutamol. NKDA.
FH	Father – HTN. MI. Mother – colon cancer.
SH	Lives with wife and children who are well. Never smoked or had alcohol.
ICE	"Is this cancer, doctor? I have a family who need me."
Dx	Tuberculosis
Ix	CXR, bloods inc FBC, CRP
Mx	Anti-TB therapy for 6 months

54M presents with cough

HPC	Cough for 3 weeks, dry non-productive, getting annoying at work and home. No diurnal variation / sputum / wheeze / SOB / chest pain / PND / orthopnoea / fever / oedema / previous episodes / weight loss / anorexia / lethargy / travel recently / coryza / itchy eyes
PMH	Recently diagnosed HTN, hay fever, leg fracture
DH	New blood pressure medication "something-pril", vitamins. NKDA
FH	Father – HTN, MI. Mother – HTN, lung cancer.
SH	Lives with wife and kids who are well. Works as priest. Non-smoker, no alcohol.
ICE	"My mother's cancer started with a cough like this…"
Dx	ACE-inhibitor intolerance
Ix	CXR
Mx	Trial off ramipril, change to ARB and monitor cough.

HAEMOPTYSIS
GENERAL FRAMEWORK

"WIPE" – Introduce yourself, whilst gaining consent
- Wash hands
- Introduce self – "Hello, my name is X and I am a medical student"
- Patient details – "Could I ask your full name and age?"
- Explain – "I have been asked to speak with you about what brings you in, would that be alright?"

Open
- Open – I understand you've coughed up blood, which I can imagine must have been very distressing. Would you mind telling me about what's happened?
- Clarify

Timeline
1. When did you start coughing up blood?
2. ~~Come on suddenly or gradually?~~
3. Does this come and go or do you have blood every time you cough?
4. Have you been coughing up blood increasingly frequently?
5. Had you ever coughed up blood like this in the past?

Symptoms
- **Blood**
  - ➢ What does the blood look like?
    - ➢ Bright-red = fresh blood
    - ➢ Rusty-brown = pneumonia
    - ➢ Frothy = HF
  - ➢ How much blood? Splatter/ Spoonfuls/ Cupfuls?
- **Sputum** – Do you cough up any sputum? How much? How often? What does it look like?
  - ➢ Purulent green/ yellow sputum = bacterial
  - ➢ Rusty sputum = pneumonia
  - ➢ Frothy white sputum with blood = pulmonary oedema
- **Risk**
  - ➢ **Illness** – Have you been ill recently?
  - ➢ **Travel** – Have you been on any long-haul flights recently? (PE) Have you travelled anywhere outside of the UK recently? (TB/ Infection)
  - ➢ **Exposure** – Is there any chance you've been exposed to asbestos/ farming/ organic dusts? (Can ask here or with SHx) (Asbestosis, cancer)
  - ➢ **Trauma** – Have you had any recent fractures? (PE)
  - ➢ **Pregnancy** – Is there any change you could be pregnant? (PE)

Systems
- **Cardiovascular** – Do you get any chest pain? Have you lost consciousness? Do you feel SOB? Do you ever get breathless lying down or at night? How many pillows do you sleep with? Have you noticed swelling in your ankles or lower back?
- **Respiratory** – Do you get any chest pain? SOB? Wheeze?
- **Constitutional** – How has your appetite been? Have you noticed a change in weight? Fevers? Night-sweats? Hoarseness/ dysphagia/ wheezing/ stridor?

ICE

- You've given me a lot of information, thank you. I'd like to hear a little about what you think could be going on. Do you have any idea?
- Is there anything that's particularly concerning you that you'd like to discuss?
- What exactly are you looking for today, resolution or reassurance?

PMHx

- Do you have any medical conditions?
- Ask a few specific questions to show that you're thinking about different causes
- Specifically, I'd like to ask if you've ever been diagnosed with:
  - ➤ Heart disease? Respiratory infections? Blood clots? Cancer? Tuberculosis? Clotting disorders?

DHx

- On any medication? Any doses of medication changed?
  - ➤ Specifically ask: OCP? Blood thinners?
- Any allergies?

FHx

- Any conditions run in the family? Specifically, I'd like to ask about asthma/ eczema/ hay-fever (atopy)? Tuberculosis? Heart problems? Lung problems? At what age? (Cystic Fibrosis/ alpha1-antitrypsin deficiency)
- Is anyone else in the family experiencing the same symptoms as you at the moment? (Infectious cause) And what about in the past? (FHx)

SHx

- SMOKING (COPD/ Malignancy)/ Alcohol/ Recreational drugs
- Home environment? Support?
- OCCUPATION (ASBESTOS?/ FARMING?)– impact on life and on occupation?

Summarise and Thank

- I'd just like to summarise back to you to make sure I haven't missed anything
- Is there anything you'd like to talk about that we haven't quite addressed?
- Thank you for talking to me and I wish you all the best

Investigations

Examination	Respiratory examination
Bedside	Oxygen saturations, temperature
Bloods	FBC, CRP, U&E, coagulation
Imaging	CXR, CT chest, CTPA or V/Q scan
Special	Bronchoscopy and biopsy, sputum MC&S, autoimmune bloods

Differential Diagnosis

	Diagnosis	Features In History	Features In Investigations	Management
ACUTE	**Pulmonary embolus**	Haemoptysis with history of pleuritic sharp chest pain, SOB. RF for PE (immobilisation, surgery, COCP, pregnant, long journey), preceding swollen painful calf, previous / FH of PE	Examination- Reduced saturations, CXR may show wedge of reduced vascularisation, ECG: most common – sinus tachycardia, (rarely S1Q3T). Raised D-dimer. Thrombus on CTPA or VQ mismatch in V/Q scan.	Anticoagulation (3 months for provoked, 6 months for unprovoked PE minimum), consider thrombophilia testing if recurrent. Thrombolysis if Haemodynamically compromised.
	Epistaxis	Coughing up blood, no sputum, no SOB, not progressive, intermittent. History of nose bleeds / rhinitis.	No chest findings, may be polyps in nose and evidence or blood or excoriations.	Reassurance for haemoptysis and investigations and management of epistaxis if problematic.
	Pneumonia	Pleuritic pain with SOB & Fever. Rust coloured sputum which can be mistaken for haemoptysis	Consolidation on CXR, raised CRP and WCC on bloods.	Empirical Antibiotics, Sputum Culture, Paracetamol
CHRONIC	**Tuberculosis**	Ongoing productive cough, weight loss, fevers, appetite loss, night sweats. Travel to endemic TB region in last year, or previous TB, no BCG vaccine.	Apical reduced air entry and crackles. CXR: apical consolidation. Bloods: raised WCC, CRP, Quantiferon positive (an IFN-y release assay [IGRA]). Early morning sputum positive for acid fast bacilli.	Commence anti-TB treatment (RIPE for 2 months then RI for 4 months). Contact precautions in hospital.
	Lung cancer	Chronic history of cough and haemoptysis, progressive shortness of breath. B-symptoms: fevers, lethargy, appetite loss, weight loss, sweats. History of smoking, FHx cancer.	May hear monophonic wheeze in bronchial cancer. Mass on CXR. CT chest – mass and lymphadenopathy.	MDT approach to consider resection vs. chemo/radiotherapy or combination. Smoking cessation.
	Bronchiectasis	Chronic histories of recurrent infections, chronic cough often with thick sputum and blood, shortness of breath. May have B-symptoms.	Coarse crackles on auscultation that change but do not go away on coughing. Area of consolidation, prominent bronchi (tram tracks) on CXR. CT Chest shows tram tracks and signet ring signs.	Respiratory physiotherapy and carbocysteine to reduce and mobilise excess sputum, aggressive antibiotics if infection, may need resection.
	Consider vasculitides e.g. Goodpasture's, Wegener's, Churg-Strauss etc. if there are symptoms of systemic illness (renal impairment/ upper respiratory tract).			

Marking Criteria Haemoptysis	Marks	
	Awarded	Available
Washes hands at the start of the station		1
Introduces themselves – Including First name, last name and role		1
Patient details confirmed: Full name, Age/ D.O.B.		1
Explains purpose of consultation		1
Open question about what brings the patient in today + Clarification of any ambiguity		1
Timeline allows a clear understanding of onset and progression - Onset/ Circumstance - ~~Sudden vs. gradual~~ - Fluctuations - Progression - Past episodes		3

Symptoms elicited are relevant and clearly directed at either arriving at a diagnosis or excluding other plausible diagnoses
- Blood
   o Appearance
   o Amount
- Sputum
- Risk – **"TIE TAP"**
   o Travel
   o Illness
   o Exposure
   o Trauma
   o Allergens
   o Pregnancy
		5

Systems queried are relevant to the complaint and adequate questions are asked for each symptom - Cardiovascular; Respiratory; Constitutional		5
Explores **Ideas, Concerns and Expectations**		3
Elicits relevant **Past Medical History** - Heart problems; Respiratory infections; Blood clot; Clotting disorder; COPD; Cancer; TB		2
Elicits relevant **Drug History** including **Allergies**		2
Elicits relevant **Family History**		2
Elicits relevant **Social History** – including Smoking/ alcohol/ recreational drugs; Home environment and support; Occupation and impact on life		2
Closes consultation appropriately allowing the patient to ask any questions		1
Presentation: structured, concise		2
Appropriate Differential Diagnosis ± Investigations ± Management Plan		3
Examiner mark – professionalism and rapport		5
Patient mark – professionalism and rapport		5

Consultation	Presentation	Global marks patient	Global marks examiner	Total
30	5	5	5	45

31F presents with coughing up blood

HPC	Has been coughing up blood for a day – bright red, sometimes stained sputum, sometimes half a teaspoon. Also has some chest pain, right sided, sharp on breathing, aching at rest, no radiation. Some shortness of breath on exertion. No fevers / lethargy / recent travel / calf pain / ill contacts / immobility.
PMH	Eczema, c-section 1 month ago
DH	Nil regular prescriptions meds, vitamins. NKDA
FH	Father – MI. Mother – rheumatoid arthritis.
SH	Lives at home with husband and 1-month old baby. Non-smoker, no alcohol.
ICE	"Am I really ill, can I pass it to my baby?"
Dx	Pulmonary embolism (provoked)
Ix	CXR then V/Q scan. Bloods incl. FBC, clotting
Mx	Anticoagulation for 3 months minimum

79M presents with chronic cough

HPC	Cough ongoing for over a month. Started gradually, cough worsening – sometimes productive of bright red blood, teaspoonful at a time. Increasing shortness of breath. Not better despite 2 courses of antibiotics and steroids. Lethargy worsening over last few months, lost his appetite and lost 8kg in last 2 months (75kg to 67kg), getting drenching night sweats occasionally – increased recently "makes me have to change my bed clothes!". No recent travel / fevers / previous TB / travel to south-east Asia / wheeze / chest pain / PND / orthopnoea / oedema / new medications.
PMH	COPD, HTN, T2DM, high cholesterol
DH	Amlodipine, ramipril, atorvastatin, metformin, gliclazide, salbutamol, symbicort. NKDA.
FH	Father – HTN. MI. Mother – pancreatic cancer.
SH	Lives alone, children are close by who help. Once a day carer for meals. Smoker 30/day for 60 years, Drinks 6 pack of beer on most weekends.
ICE	"Just can't shake this infection, can you give stronger antibiotics, doctor?"
Dx	Lung cancer
Ix	CXR then staging CT scan, bloods incl. FBC, CRP
Mx	MDT for management, counselling

71M presents with cough

HPC	Ongoing cough over last 3 months. Was non-productive for 6 weeks but came in today as noticed blood for the first time. Travelled to Pakistan to visit his family 6 months ago. Insidious onset of shortness of breath with reduced exercise tolerance. Normally sleeps easy with 2 pillows at night but recently has been feeling particularly unwell. His wife commented that his clothes are a lot sweatier in the mornings. Denies chest pain, palpitations, weight loss, loss of appetite. Had tuberculosis as a teenager when in Pakistan but did not have any further episodes.
PMH	Rheumatoid arthritis, HTN, T2DM, PE 10 years ago, Heart failure, MI x 3 with CABG 15y ago.
DH	Carvedilol, Spironolactone, Ramipril, Ranolazine, GTN Spray, Metformin. Prednisolone, Methotrexate. Infliximab infusions started a few months ago.
FH	Nil Significant
SH	Lives with wife, son, daughter in law and 2 grandchildren. Independent with good mobility.
ICE	"Is it cancer, doctor?"
Dx	Tuberculosis
Ix	CXR, Sputum Culture x 3 (or Bronchoalveolar lavage if unable) followed by Staging CT.
Mx	Refer to infectious diseases and start Combination Drugs (Rifampicin, Isoniazid, Ethambutol and Pyrinzinamide)

ABDOMINAL HISTORIES

ABDOMINAL PAIN
"WOCC SOCRATES"

<u>**"WIPE"**</u> – Introduce yourself, whilst gaining consent
- Wash hands
- Introduce self – "Hello, my name is X and I am a medical student"
- Patient details – "Could I ask your full name and age?"
- Explain – "I have been asked to speak with you about what brings you in, would that be alright?"

<u>**Open**</u>
- I understand you're suffering from pain in your tummy, can you tell me a little bit more about that?
- <u>C</u>larification
- <u>C</u>onsider pain relief – You seem to be in a lot of pain. Have you been offered pain relief?

<u>S</u>ite – Where exactly is the pain?

<u>O</u>nset
1. When did you first notice the pain? Did anything happen then?
2. Did the pain come on suddenly or gradually?
3. Does it come and go or is it always there?
4. Has the pain been getting worse?
5. Have you ever had a pain like this before?

<u>C</u>haracter – What does the pain feel like?
- E.g. Sharp stab, dull ache, colicky/ cyclical pain

<u>R</u>adiation – Does this pain go anywhere else?

<u>A</u>ssociated
- **Symptoms**
  - ➤ **Meals** – Is the pain related to meals?
  - ➤ **Fatty food** – do fatty foods make the pain worse? (Biliary colic)
  - ➤ **Jaundice** – Have you noticed any yellowing of your skin or eyes? (Cholecystitis, cholangitis)
  - ➤ **Periods** – is the pain related to your periods? (Menstrual pain)
- Systems
  - ➤ <u>**Cardiorespiratory**</u> – Have you had any chest pain? Breathlessness? Cough? ±sputum/ blood? (Pneumonia or ACS can mimic abdominal pain)
  - ➤ <u>**Gastrointestinal**</u> – How's your appetite? Swallow? Any vomiting (±blood)? How have your bowels been (diarrhoea/ constipation)? Have you noticed any changes in your stool? (mucus/ blood)
  - ➤ <u>**Genitourinary**</u> – How are the waterworks? Is the pain related to passing urine? Have you noticed any blood in your urine? Have you been going more frequently? Urgency in going? Have you been incontinent of urine?
  - ➤ <u>**Gynaecological**</u> – A more personal question. Is there any chance you could be pregnant? When was last period?
  - ➤ <u>**Constitutional**</u> – Had any weight loss? Any fevers? Any night sweats?

<u>T</u>iming - done

<u>E</u>xacerbating/ Relieving
- Does anything make the pain better?
  - ➢ E.g. Leaning forward e.g. pericarditis
- Does anything make the pain worse?
  - ➢ E.g. Food (biliary colic), breathing in (pleuritic - pneumonia)

<u>S</u>everity – How would you rate the pain on a scale of 1-10? 1 being not too bad and 10 being the worst pain imaginable.

ICE
- You've given me a lot of information, thank you. I'd like to hear a little about what you think could be going on. Do you have any idea what could be causing the pain?
- Is anything concerning you that you'd particularly like to discuss?
- Is the main thing you seek from this consultation the resolution of the pain? Or reassurance?

PMHx
- Do you have any medical conditions?
- Specifically, I'd like to ask if you've ever been diagnosed with:
  - ➢ Reflux, Gallstones, Kidney stones, IBS, IBD, Atrial fibrillation (DO NOT miss ischaemic colitis as a DDx), Previous procedures/ abdominal instrumentation

DHx
- Are you on any medication at the moment?
- Consider asking about over-the-counter or alternative/ herbal medicine
- Do you have any allergies?

FHx
- Are you aware of any conditions that run in the family?
- Has anyone in the family ever gone through anything similar to what you're going though?

SHx –
- Smoking/ Alcohol/ Recreational drugs
- Home environment? Support?
- Occupation – impact of the pain on life and on occupation?

Summarise and Thank
- I'd just like to summarise back to you to make sure I haven't missed anything
- Is there anything you'd like to talk about that we haven't quite addressed?
- Thank you for talking to me and I wish you all the best

Investigations

Examination	Full abdominal examination +/- DRE, PV exam
Bedside	Urine dip, blood glucose, pregnancy test
Bloods	FBC, U&E, LFTs, CRP, beta-HCG, amylase, lipase, lactate (ischaemic bowel), VBG, ketones,
Imaging	(Depending on DDx): AXR, erect CXR, USS abdomen, CT abdomen
Special	Oesophageal pH, urea breath test, endoscopy, gastrograffin follow through.

The Acute Abdomen

Owing to the wide range of conditions that can present with acute abdominal pain, in what is often referred to as the "acute abdomen", it is useful to narrow down your differential diagnosis based on the location of the pain. In addition, its important you can distinguish between medical and surgical cause of abdominal pain. Familiarise yourself with the conditions included in the table below:

Right Hypochondriac	Epigastrium	Left Hypochondriac
Medical: Hepatitis Pneumonia **Surgical:** Cholecystitis	**Medical:** GORD Peptic Ulcers **Surgical:** Pancreatitis Cholecystitis Thoracic AAA	**Medical:** Pneumonia Gastric Ulcer **Surgical:** Ruptured spleen
Right Flank	**Umbilical**	**Left Flank**
Medical: Pyelonephritis **Surgical:** Renal Colic Retrocaecal Appendicitis	**Surgical:** AAA Pancreatitis Diverticulitis Early Appendicitis Small Bowel Obstruction	**Medical:** Pyelonephritis **Surgical:** Renal Colic
Right Iliac Fossa	**Suprapubic**	**Left Iliac Fossa**
Medical: UTI Crohn's PID **Surgical:** Appendicitis Ureteric Colic Ovarian Torsion Ectopic Pregnancy Strangulated Hernias	**Medical:** UTI Endometriosis Crohn's and UC Acute Urinary Retention **Surgical:** Urethral Stones Large Bowel Obstruction	**Medical:** UC UTI PID **Surgical:** Diverticulitis Ureteric Colic Ovarian Torsion Ectopic Pregnancy Strangulated Hernias

Generalised

> **Surgical Causes:** Peritonitis secondary to bowel perforation & ruptures (spleen, aorta, ectopic pregnancy)
> **Common Medical Causes:** Gastroenteritis, Diabetic Ketoacidosis, Spontaneous Bacterial Peritonitis
> **Rare Medical Causes:** Henoch–Schönlein Purpura, Acute Intermittent Porphyria and Sickle Cell Crisis

---

Top Tip! Small bowel and large bowel obstruction have different causes, risk factors, investigation findings and treatment. Make sure you understand the difference

Differential Diagnosis - SURGICAL

Diagnosis	Features In History	Features In Investigations	Management
Cholecystitis	RUQ pain, especially after fatty meal, associated nausea, may be colicky, jaundice. Likely had similar pains before, self-resolving. RFs: "4 Fs" fat, female, forties, fertile	Murphy's positive on examination, guarding. Raised WCC and CRP, Raised ALP and GGT. USS shows cholecystitis or cholelithiasis	Antibiotics (ceftriaxone and Metronidazole) and planned cholecystectomy in 4-6 weeks if stable.
Appendicitis	Pain starts in umbilicus and migrates to RLQ, associated diarrhoea and fever. NB: consider mesenteric adenitis as DDx if recent viral illness and negative tests.	Very tender over McBurney's point, Rovsing positive – guarding and peritonism may be present. USS shows appendicitis. Raised WCC and CRP, raised amylase (abdominal inflammation)	Surgical opinion for intervention. IV fluids, antibiotics (ceftriaxone and Metronidazole)
Bowel Obstruction	Abdominal pain associated with constipation, obstipation, abdominal distension, nausea and vomiting. May be ileus after abdominal surgery or obstructing cancer (ask about red flags, B symptoms, previous colonoscopies)	Abdominal distension, generalised tenderness, absent or "tinkling" bowel sounds. AXR: dilated bowel loops or air under diaphragm in CXR. Gastrograffin follow through may show apple core sign in cancer.	"Drip and suck" – IV fluids, NG tube on free drainage and treat underlying cause of obstruction.
Pancreatitis	Sudden onset epigastric pain, severe, radiates to back, better leaning forward, nausea and vomiting. Most commonly history of alcohol excess, gall stones, hyperlipidaemia.	Generalised pain, no peritonism, no masses. Pyrexia and hypoxaemia. Raised amylase and lipase (more sensitive and specific), raised CRP and WCC	Score prognosis on Glasgow and Ranson's criteria, Admit, NBM and IV fluids (ITU if severe).
AAA	History of insidious back/ loin pain which may suddenly have gotten worse with new abdominal pain. May get early satiety, nausea, lower urinary tract symptoms, DVTs from local compression. Risk Factors include IDH, diabetes, family history, smoker.	Unwell patient, low blood pressure, tachycardia, pulsatile and expansile mid abdominal mass. USS to confirm. FAST scan for blood in abdomen.	ABCD! Urgent fluid resuscitation (ideally blood) and surgical involvement.
Diverticulitis	LLQ pain and diarrhoea, with fevers and rigors. Usually elderly with a history of constipation. Stool may be mixed with blood. Poor diet.	Tender LLQ, no guarding unless complications (perforation / abscess). Raised WCC and CRP.	NBM, IV fluids, ceftriaxone and Metronidazole. Re-introduce low fibre diet then long term for high fibre diet and education.
Strangulated Hernia	Abdominal pain, nausea and vomiting (feculent in late obstruction) associated with constipation, and abdominal distension. May have history of lump that usually goes back in but now stuck, tender and red. RF: Constipation, abdominal surgery, obesity.	Abdominal distension, generalised tenderness, absent or "tinkling" bowel sounds. AXR shows dilated bowel loops. (Look for perforation: Rigler's sign or air under diaphragm in erect CXR). Doppler USS: for hernia to evaluate blood flow.	"Drip and suck" – IV fluids, NG tube on free drainage and urgent surgical referral for repair.

Differential Diagnosis - UROLOGICAL

Diagnosis	Features In History	Features In Investigations	Management
Renal Colic	Sudden severe pain from "loin to groin" on one side, find it hard to get comfortable, haematuria, previous history of kidney stones. Fever and rigors may indicate pyelonephritis.	Tender over renal angle. Blood leucocytes on urine dip. USS KUB shows stone in ureter	Stones < 5mm likely pass spontaneously. >5mm likely to need urological intervention. Tamsulosin can help.
Acute Urinary Retention	Gradual onset, progressive, severe suprapubic pain with a history of not passing urine. History of BPH (nocturia, slow stream, frequency, terminal dribbling). May have recently started new drugs (anti-cholinergics), or had recent surgery.	Acutely painful suprapubically, palpable bladder, dull to percussion (mass that you can't get under). Bladder scan shows full bladder.	Urinary catheter and TWOC at later date after treating underlying cause (e.g. tamsulosin and finasteride for BPH, change of medications)
Urinary Tract Infection	Suprapubic pain associated with dysuria associated with urinary frequency, fevers, rigors. Urine may appear cloudy / bloody and be odorous. RF: Female, recent catheterisation, elderly are risk factors	Examination: suprapubic tenderness, pyrexia. Bedside: urine positive for leucocytes and nitrites. Bloods: raised WCC, CRP	Antibiotics – trimethoprim 3 days or nitrofurantoin for 5 days.

Differential Diagnosis - GYNAECOLOGICAL

Diagnosis	Features In History	Features In Investigations	Management
Ectopic Pregnancy	Gradually worsening pain in lower right/left quadrant, may have shoulder tip pain, PV bleeding and/or discharge. Last menstrual period > 4 weeks ago and sexually active, no contraceptive used. Red flags – shoulder tip pain, faintness (implies rupture)	Severe lower quadrant tenderness. Urine and blood. b-HCG positive. Red flags – haemodynamic compromise, PV bleed FAST scan for fluid in peritoneum. USS for intrauterine pregnancy.	If compromised: Immediate gynaecology consult, admit, IV fluids, cross match blood, NBM and prepare for surgery.
Ovarian Torsion or Cyst Rupture	Sudden onset right/left lower quadrant pain, constant, may have nausea and vomiting. No change in bowel or bladder habits. Previous history of ovarian pathology / PCOS.	Very tender lower quadrant, may have guarding, no mass. Adnexal tenderness on PV exam. USS pelvis shows cyst with reduced blood flow or rupture.	Analgesia, gynaecology referral.
Pelvic Inflammatory Disease	Lower abdominal pain, worsening, fevers, feeling unwell. PV discharge, deep dyspareunia, abnormal bleeding, history of STIs, risky sexual practices (no barrier protection, multiple sexual partners)	Tender in lower abdomen, usually no guarding or peritonism. PV exam – cervical excitation (perhaps adnexal tenderness), discharge present. Positive endocervical swabs	Analgesia, prolonged course of antibiotics (triple therapy) and counselling about complications of PID (sterility) and safe sexual practice.

Differential Diagnosis – MEDICAL

Diagnosis	Features In History	Features In Investigations	Management
Diabetic Ketoacidosis	Generalised abdominal pain associated with polyuria, polydipsia, nausea, vomiting, weight loss, lethargy and weakness. May have altered consciousness/ confusion, tiredness. PMH: T1DM with poor control	Look unwell, dehydrated (poor capillary refill, rapid weak pulse, low BP, dry membranes) High blood glucose level, glycosuria, ketonuria. Acidosis on blood gas Raised blood ketones	Admit. Immediate IV fluids and fixed rate insulin infusion with potassium replacement. Look for trigger (e.g. infection, MI)
Gastritis / GORD	Burning epigastric pain, worse lying down and leaning forward, worse after meals, obesity, may radiate up into chest.	CXR may show hiatus hernia. Urea breath test for *H. pylori.* Endoscopy to look for Barrett's or hiatus hernia.	Simple antacids, PPI, *H. pylori* eradication. Weight loss.
Peptic Ulcer Disease	Epigastric pain associated with GORD, chronic NSAID / corticosteroid use. Worse before meals (gastric) or after (duodenal). May get vomiting with moderate amounts of fresh red blood or "coffee grounds" in vomit.	Examination: epigastric tenderness, blood in vomit. Positive urea breath test. Ulcer on endoscopy.	*H. pylori* eradication and PPI therapy. If haematemesis: admit, inpatient endoscopy, may need intervention if actively bleeding.
IBD	Generalised abdominal pain associated with frequent, intermittent, chronic, loose stools (may be bloody / have mucous), weight loss, anorexia, lethargy. Extra intestinal: eyes, joint pains, skin rashes, perianal abscess.	Generalised abdominal tenderness, may have RIF mass (ileocecal) Raised WCC, CRP. Faecal calprotectin raised. AXR may show thumb printing. Colonoscopy for biopsy (?transmural inflammation)	Rehydrate, immunosuppression (prednisolone, azathioprine, infliximab etc. depending on response)
Gastroenteritis	Sudden onset, generalised pain, diarrhoea and vomiting with urgency, sick contacts or close living quarters (halls / nursing home / recent admission), fever, myalgia, lethargy.	Raised WCC and CRP may be present. Positive stool cultures if parasitic / bacterial.	Usually viral and self-terminating.
Hepatitis	RUQ pain, fever, jaundice, malaise and return from endemic country for Hepatitis A – faeco oral risk factors (street food, non-filtered water). Hepatitis B – travel to endemic areas. Preceded by vomiting and fever.	Exam: jaundice, dehydration from vomiting. Bloods: abnormal LFTs, raised bilirubin. Positive serology for viral hepatitis.	Acute Hep A & B: Self-limiting, supportive treatment. Chronic Hep B: Antivirals, monitor for HCC. Hep C: interferon therapy in acute and antivirals in chronic.
Spontaneous Bacterial Peritonitis	Severe pain and unwell patient with history of chronic liver disease and ascites. Fevers, encephalopathy, diarrhoea, ileus.	Exam: tender ascitic abdomen, may have rebound and guarding. Signs of chronic liver disease. Bloods: deranged LFTs Ascitic tap: raised protein, raised WCC	Admit, empirical antibiotic therapy after ascitic tap (e.g. IV cefotaxime) until MC&S known.

Marking Criteria ABDOMINAL PAIN	Marks	
	Awarded	Available
Washed hands at the start of the station		1
Introduced themselves – Including First name, last name and role		1
Patient details confirmed: Full name, Age/ D.O.B.		1
Explained purpose of consultation		1
Open question about what brings the patient in today + Clarification of any ambiguity		1
Site – Enquires about exact location of abdominal pain		1
Onset (Timeline) – Asks questions to provide a clear understanding of onset and progression - Onset/ Circumstance - Sudden vs. gradual - Fluctuations - Progression - Past episodes		3
Character - Obtains an accurate description of the abdominal pain (Ex. Stab, ache, colic, etc.)		1
Radiation - Asks about the pain moving anywhere else		1
Associated symptoms ■ **Symptoms** elicited are relevant and clearly directed at either arriving at a diagnosis or excluding other plausible diagnoses - Meals - Fatty food - Jaundice - Periods ■ **Systems** queried are relevant to the complaint and adequate questions are asked for each symptom - Cardiorespiratory; Gastrointestinal; Genitourinary; Gynaecological; Constitutional		6
Timing - This has been done		0
Exacerbation/ Relief - Clearly asks if the patient has noticed any relieving/ exacerbating factors, providing appropriate examples if prompted (Ex. Food; breathing; sitting forwards)		1
Severity - Subjective quantitative assessment of chest pain severity		1
Explores **Ideas, Concerns and Expectations**		3
Elicits relevant **Past Medical History** - Reflux; Gallstones; Kidney stones; IBS; IBD; AF; Previous procedures/ abdominal instrumentation		2
Elicits relevant **Drug History** including **Allergies**		2
Elicits relevant **Family History**		2
Elicits relevant **Social History** – including Smoking/ alcohol/ recreational drugs; **Home** environment and support; **Occupation** and impact on life		2
Closes consultation appropriately allowing the patient to ask any questions		1
Presentation: structured, concise		2
Appropriate Differential Diagnosis ± Investigations ± Management Plan		3
Examiner mark – professionalism and rapport		5
Patient mark – professionalism and rapport		5

Consultation	Presentation	Global marks patient	Global marks examiner	Total
30	5	5	5	45

35F presents with abdominal pain

HPC	1 day of abdominal pain, started in the middle /generalised but now is more on the lower right side of the abdomen, now 8/10, not radiating anywhere, associated with nausea and vomiting, has had 2x loose stools (no blood or mucous), feeling feverish for the last 2 hours, not wanting to eat. No relieving factors. Pressing on RIF makes it worse. Was well before this. No abdominal distension / ill contacts / travel / previous episodes / associated with new food / dysphagia / odynophagia / haematemesis / chance of pregnancy
PMH	GORD, rotator cuff injury
DH	Omeprazole, paracetamol, combined contraceptive pill. NKDA.
FH	Father - Colon cancer
SH	Lives with partner who is well. Social smoker 10/week, 6 pints at weekends. No drugs.
ICE	"Please make the pain better!"
Dx	Appendicitis
Ix	USS abdomen, bloods incl. FBC, CRP, lactate and lipase, erect CXR to rule out perforation
Mx	Analgesia, nil by mouth, IV fluids, surgical referral.

57F presents with abdominal pain

HPC	Abdominal pain started 3 hours ago after dinner (fried chicken and chips), top middle and right of tummy, 7/10 pain, sometimes comes and goes in waves, but is also there all the time, nothing helps the pain. Has had pain before, usually after meals (especially after fish and chips) – on and off for the last 6 months. Felt a bit sweaty today with nausea, but no fevers. Does think her skin looks more yellow. No rigors / weight loss ("I wish!") / fevers / lethargy / diarrhoea / vomiting / dysphagia / change in bowel habit / blood in stool / abdominal distension / alcohol excess / previous liver disease
PMH	T2DM, obesity (BMI = 38), hysterectomy, osteoarthritis
DH	Metformin, gliclazide, paracetamol, codeine. NKDA
FH	Mother – diabetes, hysterectomy. Father – MI.
SH	Lives alone. Works as receptionist. Smokes 10/day, 25 years. One glass of wine a day.
ICE	"Is it my liver, because of all the wine?"
Dx	Biliary colic on a background of cholecystitis
Ix	Bloods incl. LFTs, CRP, FBC. USS abdomen, ?MRCP
Mx	Analgesia, antibiotics (ceftriaxone and metronidazole), nil by mouth, IV fluids, surgical referral

23M presents with abdominal pain

HPC	Abdominal pain for the last 6 hours, generalised in abdomen, worsening steadily, now 7/10 pain. Has had nausea and vomiting (2 times, no blood, no bile), no diarrhoea. Feeling very unwell, tired, drowsy, reduced appetite. Has had a chest infection over the last few days – productive cough, fevers, and lethargy. Poor appetite - not eating and drinking much. Feels very thirsty, but also passing lots of urine.
PMH	T1DM since age 9, asthma
DH	Insulin (novomix BD) – has been taking it if he eats, salbutamol. Allergic to penicillin.
FH	Father and sister- diabetes
SH	Works as mechanic. Lives alone. Smoker, 15/day for 5 years. Social alcohol – 5 pints at weekends.
ICE	"I was thinking it might be appendicitis, do I need surgery?"
Dx	Diabetic Ketoacidosis
Ix	Blood glucose, ketones and gas to look at pH, urinalysis, bloods incl. FBC, U&E
Mx	Aggressive IV rehydration, fixed rate insulin, potassium replacement, regular blood glucose and neuro observations, treat underlying cause (intercurrent infection) – HDU care ideally.

45 year old male with abdominal pain and generally unwell

HPC	Patient reports 1 week history of chills, nausea and vomiting. Reports fevers and night sweats. Reports abdominal pain and loss of appetite. Patient does not report any dizziness or SOB. No chest pain. No cough or colds. Patient reports some dysuria. Patient describes worsening abdominal distension and weight gain. Also reports some leg swelling over last two months.
PMH	Hepatitis B
DH	NKDA, Tenofovir
FHx	Nil relevant
SH	50 units alcohol per week, current smoker. Ex-IVDU.
ICE	"Doctor, this pain is really worrying me. I'm afraid my Tenofovir isn't working anymore."
Dx	Spontaneous Bacterial Peritonitis
Ix	FBC, U&E, LFT, CRP, blood cultures, aspiration and culture of ascitic fluid, USS liver, vitamin B and folate
Mx	Antibiotics, consider ascitic tab in case large amount of ascites present, alcohol and smoking cessation advice, refer to community alcohol team

25 year old female with abdominal pain

HPC	Patient presents with gradual onset abdominal pain. Pain limited to right iliac fossa but radiating to mid line and epigastric region. Patient says pain started 1 week ago and has gradually been getting worse. She describes no distension in her abdomen. Patient reports no nausea or vomiting. Some diarrhoea and dysuria. No headaches, no dizziness, no palpitations. Patient does not report any fevers.
PMH	Chlamydia infection 2 years ago, treated with antibiotics. Not on contraception.
DH	NKDA, nil regular
FH	Nil relevant
SH	Long term boy friend, drinks 20 units of alcohol per week. Non-smoker.
ICE	"I can't handle this pain anymore doctor. Can't you please give me some pain relief?"
Dx	Ectopic pregnancy
Ix	Pregnancy test, USS pelvis, FBC, U&E, LFT, CRP, β-hCG
Mx	Treatment choice depends on urgency of treatment. Methotrexate or surgical removal of pregnancy and likely associated Fallopian tube.

Top Tip! Remember that many of the presentations above can lead to organ rupture (appendix, colon, aorta etc.) which can then lead to signs of peritonism: rigid abdomen, pain exacerbated by any movement. Similarly bowel obstruction due to cancer, volvulus, adhesions or strangulated hernias may lead to intestinal perforation which presents in a similar manner.

Signs of peritonism on examination: guarding, rigidity, rebound tenderness. These patients are a surgical emergency and require immediate surgical review and potentially prepping for urgent surgery.

DYSPHAGIA
GENERAL FRAMEWORK

"WIPE" – Introduce yourself, whilst gaining consent
- Wash hands
- Introduce self – "Hello, my name is X and I am a medical student"
- Patient details – "Could I ask your full name and age?"
- Explain – "I have been asked to speak with you about what brings you in, would that be alright?"

Open
- I understand you've had problems with your swallowing, would you mind telling me more about that?
- **Clarify** – Before you tell me some more, it's important for me just to ask whether you struggle with swallowing solids, liquids or both?

Timeline
1. When did you start having swallowing problems? Did anything happen then?
2. Did it come on suddenly or gradually? Did it start with solids, liquids or both?
3. Do these swallow problems come and go or are they always there?
4. Have they been getting worse?
5. Have you ever had swallowing problems before?

Symptoms – Remember as: "MPS ROB"
1. **Motion** – Do you find it difficult to **initiate** the swallow or **swallowing** itself?
2. **Pain** – Do you have any **pain** when you swallow?
3. **Smell** – Have you noticed bad breath recently?
4. **Regurgitation** – Do you ever **bring up** food or drink after you've swallowed?
5. **hOarseness** – Have you noticed any **hoarseness** in your voice?
6. **Bulging/ Gargling** – any **bulging** of neck or **gargling** on eating?

Systems
- **Neurological** – Have you had a headache? Noticed a change in any of your senses? Any weakness? Odd sensations? Is it more difficult to swallow at the end of a meal? (myasthenia)
- **Gastrointestinal** – How has your appetite been? Have you been sick at all? ±Blood Have you had any tummy pain? Have you noticed a change in bowel habit? A more personal question. Have you noticed any change in your stool?
- **Anxiety** – have you been feeling particularly anxious recently?
- **Dermatological** – Any skin changes? (Specifically for CREST)
- **Constitutional** – How has your appetite been? Have you noticed a change in weight? Have you been feeling tired recently? Have you had a fever? Night-sweats?

ICE
- You've given me a lot of information, thank you. I'd like to hear a little about what you think could be going on. Do you have any idea?
- Is there anything that's particularly concerning you that you'd like to discuss?
- What exactly are you looking for today, resolution or reassurance?

PMHx
- Do you have any medical conditions?
- Ask a few specific questions to show that you're thinking about different causes
- Specifically, I'd like to ask if you've ever been diagnosed with:
  - ➢ Diabetes? High BP? Heart problems like atrial Fibrillation? A stroke or something called a transient ischaemic attack? Cancer? Nervous system disease? Muscle disease?

DHx

- On any medication? Any doses of medication changed?
  - ➢ Any medication for osteoporosis?
- Any allergies?

FHx

- Any conditions in the family?
  - ➢ Cancer? Nervous system disorders? Muscle disease?
- Has anyone in the family experienced swallowing problems similar to the ones you're experiencing now?

SHx

- Smoking/ Alcohol/ Recreational drugs
- Home environment? Support?
- Occupation – impact on life and on occupation?

Summarise and Thank

- I'd just like to summarise back to you to make sure I haven't missed anything
- Is there anything you'd like to talk about that we haven't quite addressed?
- Thank you for talking to me and I wish you all the best

Investigations

Examination	Full GI and respiratory examination (signs of aspiration pneumonia in right mid zone)
Bedside	Urea breath test for *H. pylori*
Bloods	FBC (?anaemia), U&E, CRP, iron studies
Imaging	CXR, Barium swallow
Special	Oesophageal manometry, endoscopy

Differential Diagnosis

	Diagnosis	Features In History	Features In Investigations	Management
NEUROLOGICAL	**Achalasia**	Solids and liquids (but solids > soft), feels like it gets stuck, painful, and have to drink a lot of water. Regurgitation occurs, relieves pain.	Little on examination. CXR may show dilated oesophagus. Birds beak on barium swallow. Manometry of oesophagus shows increased pressure.	Medical: CCBs and nitrates to relax lower oesophagus. Sphincter. Surgical: Heller myotomy
	Myasthenia Gravis	Difficulty swallowing especially towards the end of the day or meal. Other weakness, ptosis, diplopia. Progressive. Other autoimmune conditions.	No structural findings, fatigability of repetitive movements. Anti-AChR, anti-MUSK on bloods. Positive ice test on ptosis.	Anti-cholinesterase therapy, Immunosuppression. Neurology follow up.
	Oesophageal spasm	Gripping/stabbing pain in central chest associated with dysphagia and reflux symptoms.	Endoscopy is clear of obstruction. Barium swallow may show corkscrew pattern / rosary beads. Manometry is diagnostic.	Medical: Nitrates, CCBs Interventional: Botox injection, balloon dilation.
STRUCTURAL	**Pharyngeal pouch**	Difficulty swallowing associated with lump in back of neck, bad breath, gurgling sounds and progressive worsening. May have chronic cough and weight loss.	Avoid endoscopy (may perforate lesion). Barium swallow may show outpouching.	Surgical – depending on size. Dohlman's procedure if small (opens up pouch) Diverticulectomy if large – closes defect.
	Stricture / webs	Progressive worsening of dysphagia starting with solids and progressing to softer foods. history of GORD. Ass. with autoimmune diseases (RA, thyroid, psoriasis etc.). Webs may be ass. with Fe deficiency.	Fe deficiency anaemia in Plummer-Vinson Syndrome. Barium swallow to show stricture, endoscopy to biopsy.	Medical: PPIs Interventional: Dilatation at endoscopy. Screen and safety net for aspiration pneumonitis.
	Oesophageal cancer	Progressive dysphagia (solids → liquids), vomiting, anorexia, weight loss, signs of GI bleed. B symptoms. RF: smoking, GORD (Barret's → adenocarcinoma).	"Apple core" on barium swallow. Iron deficiency.	Primarily surgical – endoscopic resection or oesophagectomy if advanced. May use radio- / chemo-adjunct.

Marking Criteria Dysphagia	Marks	
	Awarded	Available
Washes hands at the start of the station		1
Introduces themselves – Including First name, last name and role		1
Patient details confirmed: Full name, Age/ D.O.B.		1
Explains purpose of consultation		1
Open question about what brings the patient in today + Clarification of any ambiguity – clarifies whether the patient struggles with solids/ liquids/ both		1
Timeline allows a clear understanding of onset and progression - Onset/ Circumstance - ~~Sudden vs. gradual~~ - Fluctuations - Progression - Past episodes		3

Symptoms elicited are relevant and clearly directed at either arriving at a diagnosis or excluding other plausible diagnoses
- "MPS ROB"
   o Motion
   o Pain
   o Smell
   o Regurgitation
   o hOarseness
   o Bulging/ gargling
		5

Systems queried are relevant to the complaint and adequate questions are asked for each symptom - Neurological; Gastrointestinal; Anxiety; Dermatological; Constitutional		5
Explores **Ideas, Concerns and Expectations**		3
Elicits relevant **Past Medical History** - DM; HTN; Heart problems; Previous stroke or TIA; Cancer; Nervous system disease; Muscle disease		2
Elicits relevant **Drug History** including **Allergies**		2
Elicits relevant **Family History**		2
Elicits relevant **Social History** – including Smoking/ alcohol/ recreational drugs; **H**ome environment and support; **O**ccupation and impact on life		2
Closes consultation appropriately allowing the patient to ask any questions		1
Presentation: structured, concise		2
Appropriate Differential Diagnosis ± Investigations ± Management Plan		3
Examiner mark – professionalism and rapport		5
Patient mark – professionalism and rapport		5

Consultation	Presentation	Global marks patient	Global marks examiner	Total
30	5	5	5	45

51M presents with difficulty eating

HPC	Trouble swallowing for 2 months now. Initially was with big sticky things like potatoes, but gotten worse and worse over time and now is having trouble swallowing yoghurts and pureed foods. Has been constantly there, doesn't come and go. Feels like food is getting stuck half way down his chest. Helps if he drinks water afterwards to get it moving. Has not been feeling well in himself whilst this has been happening, not been able to eat much, lost 9kg in weight (was 82kg 2 months ago) and so feeling very tired in himself as well – not been going to his pub to play darts for the last week, normally every day. No weakness / progression of weakness with a meal / regurgitation / gurgling / halitosis / vomiting / cough / rashes / fevers / myalgia or arthralgia / difficulties speaking / drooling.
PMH	COPD, depression, anxiety, GORD
DH	Symbicort, tiotropium, salbutamol, Ramipril, pantoprazole, sertraline, diazepam PRN. NKDA
FH	Father – lung cancer. Mother – AF.
SH	Lives alone. Smoker, 20/day for 40 years. 6 pints of beer a night.
ICE	"It feels all closed up, can you open up again?"
Dx	Oesophageal cancer
Ix	Endoscopy, staging CT
Mx	MDT management with surgery / chemotherapy / radiotherapy / combination therapy based on stage.

48F presents with difficulty swallowing

HPC	Difficulty with swallowing for 6 months, intermittent, feels like food gets stuck in chest and then if she drinks a lot of water resolves. Solids and liquids equally and from the beginning. Sometimes gets some regurgitation. Causes pain in the chest at times – no radiation, achey, 3/10, resolves with time/ lots of water, worse on eating more at the time. Has noted more heartburn recently. Been put off food as scared if that will happen. No gurgling / neck lump / halitosis / weight loss / lethargy / fevers / night sweats / nausea / vomiting / diarrhoea / abdominal pain / weakness / difficulty initiating swallow
PMH	Hypothyroidism, GORD
DH	Levothyroxine, omeprazole. Allergic to tramadol – gets vomiting.
FH	Mother – hypothyroidism. Father – colorectal cancer.
SH	Lives with 3 cats. Non-smoker, 1 glass of wine a night.
ICE	"I'm scared the pain is to do with my heart, what if something happens?"
Dx	Achalasia
Ix	CXR, barium swallow (oesophageal dilatation with bird's beak end), endoscopy, perhaps oesophageal manometry
Mx	Young and fit – Heller myotomy, unfit for surgery - pneumonic dilatation. CCBs or nitrates if unsuitable for either.

81M presents with problems after eating

HPC	For a few months has been having problems with swallowing foods properly. Has been getting some food coming back up and has been eating a lot let because of this. Has noted a strange sound sometimes when trying to swallow. Wife complains of bad breath more in the last month. No fevers but has been having a cough for the last 2 months – dry cough, throaty, no sputum, no blood, no shortness of breath. No progression of symptoms / no lethargy / no weight loss / sweats / previous episodes.
PMH	HTN, hypercholesterolaemia, AF, arthritis
DH	Ramipril, amlodipine, simvastatin, warfarin, co-codamol
FH	Father had MI
SH	Lives with wife. Ex-smoker of 20/day for 30 years. No alcohol
ICE	"I just want to be able to eat again"
Dx	Pharyngeal pouch
Ix	CXR (look for aspiration pneumonia) Barium swallow
Mx	Diverticulotomy or Dohlman's procedure.

VOMITING
GENERAL FRAMEWORK

"WIPE" – Introduce yourself, whilst gaining consent
- Wash hands
- Introduce self – "Hello, my name is X and I am a medical student"
- Patient details – "Could I ask your full name and age?"
- Explain – "I have been asked to speak with you about what brings you in, would that be alright?"

Open
- I understand you've been vomiting recently, would you mind telling me what happened?
- Clarify – This might sound like an odd question but can I just clarify that this vomiting has been non-intentional?

Timeline
1. When did you start vomiting? What were you doing at the time?
2. Did it come on suddenly or gradually?
3. Have you been vomiting all the time or does it come and go?
4. Has it been getting worse?
5. Have you ever had anything like this before?

Symptoms
- **Vomit** – Can you describe the vomit? Is there a faecal scent? Green colour?
- **Blood** – Do you bring up any blood with the vomit?
- **Nausea** – Is this vomiting associated with a feeling of nausea?
- **Pain** – Do you experience any pain with this vomiting?
- **Food** – Had you eaten anything recently before the vomiting? What about over the last couple of days/ weeks – anything exotic? Does the vomiting always follow eating?
- **Trauma** – Have you had any trauma to your head in the last few weeks/ months?

Systems
- **Neurological** – Any headaches? A change in any of your senses? Weakness? Weird sensation anywhere in your body?
- **Gastrointestinal** – How has your appetite been? Have you had any problems swallowing? Have you had any tummy pain? Have you noticed a change in bowel habit? A more personal question. Have you noticed any change in your stool?
- **Genitourinary** – How have the waterworks been? Have you been passing urine more frequently? Increased amounts?
- **Gynaecological** – Are you sexually active? Is there any chance you could be pregnant? When was your last menstrual period?
- **Psychiatric** – How has your mood been? Have you been feeling particularly anxious recently?
- **Constitutional** – How has your appetite been? Have you noticed a change in weight? Have you been feeling tired recently? Have you had a fever? Night-sweats?

ICE
- You've given me a lot of information, thank you. I'd like to hear a little about what you think could be going on. Do you have any idea?
- Is there anything that's particularly concerning you that you'd like to discuss?
- What exactly are you looking for today, resolution or reassurance?

PMHx
- Do you have any medical conditions?
- Ask a few specific questions to show that you're thinking about different causes
- Specifically, I'd like to ask if you've ever been diagnosed with:
  - Diabetes? Something called an autoimmune disease? Complicated pregnancies? Cancer? Liver disease? Alcohol-related problems?

DHx
- On any medication? Any doses of medication changed?
- Specifically, I'd like to ask whether you're on
  - Cancer medication?

FHx
- Any conditions run in the family? Specifically, I'd like to ask about Cancer? Liver problems? Bowel problems? Eating disorders?
- Has anyone in the family ever been affected by vomiting similar to what you're describing to me now?

SHx –
- Smoking/ Alcohol/ Recreational drugs
- Home environment? Support?
- Occupation – impact on life and on occupation?

Summarise and Thank
- I'd just like to summarise back to you to make sure I haven't missed anything
- Is there anything you'd like to talk about that we haven't quite addressed?
- Thank you for talking to me and I wish you all the best

Investigations

Examination	Abdominal examination, assess fluid status for dehydration
Bedside	Urine dip, BP and HR, temperature, blood glucose
Bloods	FBC, U&E, CRP, LFTs
Imaging	AXR (?obstruction)
Special	CT abdomen

Differential Diagnosis

	Diagnosis	Features In History	Features In Investigations	Management
INFECTIVE	**Gastroenteritis**	Sudden onset, diarrhoea and vomiting, urgency, sick contacts or close living quarters (halls / nursing home / recent admission), fever, myalgia, lethargy	Raised WCC and CRP may be present	Usually viral and self-terminating.
	Food poisoning	Stereotypical time after food (6 – 24 hours after) – reheated rice / raw meat / canned food. May be associated with severe dehydration – ask about faintness, postural symptoms.	Usually nil	Supportive treatment – anti-emetics, rehydration if compromised.
SURGICAL	**Bowel obstruction**	Nausea and vomiting (faeculent in late obstruction) associated with constipation, obstipation, abdominal distension, Abdominal pain. May be ileus after abdominal surgery or obstructing cancer (ask about red flags, B symptoms, previous colonoscopies)	Abdominal distension, generalised tenderness, absent or "tinkling" bowel sounds. AXR: dilated bowel loops, perhaps fluid levels. (Look for perforation: Rigler's sign or air under diaphragm in erect CXR). Gastrograffin follow through may show apple core sign in cancer.	"Drip and suck" – IV fluids, NG tube on free drainage and treat underlying cause of obstruction.
METABOLIC	**Hyperemesis gravidarum**	Severe intractable vomiting, dehydration in the first and second trimester. No distension, diarrhoea, fevers, travel or abnormal foods. Ask about baby's health and if breastfeeding.	Usually nil – may have reduced urine output, increased urine specific gravity, raised urea and creatinine.	Rehydrate if compromised. Advice re: hydration and conservative measures to ease nausea (small meals, avoid triggers etc.). Anti-emetics (check if safe when breastfeeding)
	Diabetic Ketoacidosis	Nausea & vomiting associated with polyuria, polydipsia, generalised abdominal pain weight loss, lethargy and weakness. May have altered consciousness/ confusion, tiredness. PMH: T1DM with poor control	Look unwell, dehydrated (poor capillary refill, rapid weak pulse, low BP, dry membranes) High blood glucose level, glucosuria, ketonuria. Acidosis on blood gas Raised blood ketones	Admit. Immediate IV fluids and fixed rate insulin infusion with potassium replacement. Look for trigger (e.g. infection, MI)

Rarer Causes include: Addison's disease (following abrupt steroid cessation), eating disorders (bulimia) and raised ICP (associated with headaches).

Marking Criteria Vomiting	Marks	
	Awarded	Available
Washes hands at the start of the station		1
Introduces themselves – Including First name, last name and role		1
Patient details confirmed: Full name, Age/ D.O.B.		1
Explains purpose of consultation		1
Open question about what brings the patient in today + Clarification of any ambiguity – may confirm whether vomiting has been non-intentional (i.e.: not induced)		1

Timeline allows a clear understanding of onset and progression
  - Onset/ Circumstance
  - Sudden vs. gradual
  - Fluctuations
  - Progression
  - Past episodes
		3

Symptoms elicited are relevant and clearly directed at either arriving at a diagnosis or excluding other plausible diagnoses
  - Vomit
  - Blood
  - Nausea
  - Pain
  - Food
  - Trauma
		5

Systems queried are relevant to the complaint and adequate questions are asked for each symptom - Neurological; Gastrointestinal; Genitourinary; Gynaecological; Psychiatric; Constitutional		5
Explores **Ideas, Concerns and Expectations**		3
Elicits relevant **Past Medical History** - DM; Autoimmunity; Heart problems; Complicated pregnancies; Cancer; Liver disease; Alcohol-related problems		2
Elicits relevant **Drug History** including **Allergies**		2
Elicits relevant **Family History**		2
Elicits relevant **Social History** – including Smoking/ alcohol/ recreational drugs; **H**ome environment and support; **O**ccupation and impact on life		2
Closes consultation appropriately allowing the patient to ask any questions		1
Presentation: structured, concise		2
Appropriate Differential Diagnosis ± Investigations ± Management Plan		3
Examiner mark – professionalism and rapport		5
Patient mark – professionalism and rapport		5

Consultation	Presentation	Global marks patient	Global marks examiner	Total
30	5	5	5	45

19M presents with new onset Vomiting

HPC	Vomiting for 5 hours that woke him up from sleep. Vomit – 10-15 times, initially just food and now clear liquid and dry retching. No blood, no dark green (bile), no coffee grounds. Not able to keep anything down even water. Felt well yesterday. Had cereal for breakfast, supermarket meal deal for lunch and some left over Chinese food for dinner, not unusual for him – nothing new. Opened bowels in the evening, normal, not hard to pass or loose stool. No fevers / recent travel / ill contacts / diarrhoea / excessive wind / abdominal pain / trauma to head
PMH	Eczema
DH	Emollients, hydrocortisone cream. Allergic: penicillin
FH	Brother - Asthma, mother - colon cancer
SH	University student, smokes socially 5/week, 30 units/week
ICE	"I feel awful, I just want it to stop"
Dx	Gastroenteritis (bacillus cereus)
Ix	Examination, BP, heart rate (?dehydrated)
Mx	Anti-emetics, IV fluids to rehydrate

72M presents with worsening Vomiting

HPC	Vomiting for 2 hours but has been feeling unwell for a week and abdominal pain for 2 days. Vomit – started as nausea 1-day ago and has been worsening, vomited 6-7 times, just yellow liquid, no blood, no bile. Last one looked browner. Abdominal pain – was intermittent, now constant, started gradually, worsening, now 7/10, generalised. Has been feeling lethargic for a week, lost his appetite, especially last few days. Bowels last opened 10 days ago, had been getting harder to pass leading up to then. Tummy does seem bigger, feels bloated. Not passed wind for 1 day. No fevers / weight loss / foreign travel / ill contacts / change in diet / recent illnesses / history of cancer / recent surgery
PMH	AF, hypertension, type-2 diabetes
DH	Warfarin, amlodipine, metformin, gliclazide. Allergic: morphine
FH	Nil
SH	Lives with wife who has MS, independent ADLs, ex-smoker (20/day for 40 years), no alcohol
ICE	"I don't think I can look after my wife any more like this..."
Dx	Bowel obstruction
Ix	AXR, serum lactate (?ischaemic bowel with AF)
Mx	NBM, NG tube, IV fluids, surgical referral

37M presents with Vomiting

HPC	History of vomiting over several months. Patient also reports some diarrhoea, headache, weight loss and anxiety. Increased pigmentation on palmar crease, marked darkening of scars on forearm. Patient says he sustained them when gardening not too long ago. Says he feels dizzy and light headed. He also finds it hard to concentrate and slurs his speech.
PMH	Dizziness, especially when getting up quickly, Hashimoto's, T1DM
DH	Insulin, Levothyroxine
FH	Mother had T1DM
SH	Lives alone, ex-smoker, 4 units of alcohol per day
ICE	I need to stop vomiting, I can't keep any food down and am just always getting so dizzy.
Dx	Addison's Disease
Ix	FBC, U&E, CRP, Bone profile, synacthen test
Mx	Cortisol replacement with oral hydrocortisone or prednisolone, regular monitoring

HAEMATEMESIS
GENERAL FRAMEWORK

"WIPE" – Introduce yourself, whilst gaining consent
- Wash hands
- Introduce self – "Hello, my name is X and I am a medical student"
- Patient details – "Could I ask your full name and age?"
- Explain – "I have been asked to speak with you about what brings you in, would that be alright?"

Open
- I understand you've vomited some blood which must have been very distressing, would you mind telling me what happened?
- Clarify – Can I briefly ask you for a rough estimate of how much blood?

(At this point inform the examiner this could be a medical emergency and that you would want to calculate a pre-endoscopy Blatchford or Rockall score and escalate accordingly. Then return to your history)

Timeline
1. When did you start vomiting blood? What were you doing at the time?
2. Did it come on suddenly or gradually?
3. Have you been vomiting all the time or does it come and go?
4. Has it been getting worse?
5. Have you ever had anything like this before?

Symptoms
- **Blood** – Is the blood bright-red or dark like "coffee grounds"?
- **Pain** – Did you experience any pain with this bleed?
- **Vomit** – Do you bring up any vomit? (If yes) Is the blood mixed in with the vomit or at the beginning/ end?
- **Reflux** – Do you suffer from reflux?
- **Trauma** – Have you recently ingested anything that could have damaged your food-pipe? Have you had any procedures done recently?
- **"RA" – Retching/ Alcohol binge** – had you been retching beforehand? Recent alcohol binge?

Systems
- **Gastrointestinal** – How has your appetite been? Have you had any problems swallowing? Have you had any tummy pain? Have you noticed a change in bowel habit? A more personal question. Have you noticed any change in your stool?
- **Constitutional** – How has your appetite been? Have you noticed a change in weight? Have you been feeling tired recently? Have you had a fever? Night-sweats?

ICE
- You've given me a lot of information, thank you. I'd like to hear a little about what you think could be going on. Do you have any idea?
- Is there anything that's particularly concerning you that you'd like to discuss?
- What exactly are you looking for today, resolution or reassurance?

PMHx
- Do you have any medical conditions?
- Ask a few specific questions to show that you're thinking about different causes
- Specifically, I'd like to ask if you've ever been diagnosed with:
  - ➤ Bleeding disorder? Peptic ulcer disease or tummy varices? Cancer? Liver disease? Have you had procedures (endoscopy) done recently? Alcohol-related problems?

DHx

- On any medication? Any doses of medication changed?
- Specifically, I'd like to ask whether you're on
  - ➢ Blood thinning medication? (Aspirin? Anticoagulants?) Anti-inflammatory drugs? Painkillers? (Aspirin? Ibuprofen? Diclofenac?) Steroids? Warfarin?

FHx

- Any conditions run in the family? Specifically, I'd like to ask about bleeding disorders? Cancer? Alcoholism?
- Has anyone in the family ever been affected by something similar to what you're describing to me?

SHx

- Smoking/ Alcohol/ Recreational drugs
- Home environment? Support?
- Occupation – impact on life and on occupation?

Summarise and Thank

- I'd just like to summarise back to you to make sure I haven't missed anything
- Is there anything you'd like to talk about that we haven't quite addressed?
- Thank you for talking to me and I wish you all the best

Investigations

Examination	Abdominal examination, DRE
Bedside	BP, HR, temperature, urinalysis
Bloods	FBC, U&E, clotting, LFTs
Imaging	AXR, CT chest and abdomen
Special	Endoscopy, urea breath test, barium swallow

Differential Diagnosis

	Diagnosis	Features In History	Features In Investigations	Management
OESOPHAGEAL	**Variceal Bleed**	Large amount of fresh red blood in vomit, abdominal pain. History of chronic liver disease, alcohol excess, other causes of portal hypertension.	May be Haemodynamically compromised, reduced GCS, septic. Endoscopy – bleeding varices or clotted site of bleed.	Fluid resuscitation (ideally with blood), terlipressin, prophylactic antibiotics, variceal ligation. TIPSS if uncontrollable bleed.
	Mallory-Weiss	Small amounts of fresh red blood in vomitus after a history of vomiting/ retching a lot in a short period of time, some pain, dizziness. Ensure no history of nose / gum bleed that they may have swallowed.	May be dehydrated due to vomiting, only small amounts of fresh red blood. No physical signs.	Most mucosal tears heal quickly, endoscopy is diagnostic but often not necessary unless large amounts or unwell patient.
GASTRIC	**Gastric Cancer**	Anorexia, early satiety, weight loss, dyspepsia and lethargy with haematemesis. RF: smoking, elderly, east Asian, FHx, pernicious anaemia.	Exam – may have epigastric mass Blood – iron deficiency anaemia Barium swallow may delineate mass. Endoscopy and biopsy to diagnose.	Surgical resection with perioperative combination chemotherapy (5-FU).
	Peptic Ulcer	Moderate amounts of fresh red blood or "coffee grounds" in vomit. Associated with history of epigastric pain, GORD, chronic NSAID / corticosteroid use.	Examination: blood in vomit, epigastric tenderness. Bloods: may show dehydration (raised urea and creatinine) Ulcer on endoscopy.	Admit and inpatient endoscopy, may need intervention if actively bleeding. *H. pylori* eradication and PPI therapy.

Also consider: Oesophageal cancer and iatrogenic damage during endoscopy

Top Tip! Remember to quote pre-endoscopy Rockall and Blatchford scores when asked how you would manage a patient with haematemesis:

Rockall	1	2	≥ 3
Blatchford	0	< 4	≥ 6
Action	Early discharge	Unlikely to need urgent endoscopy	Urgent endoscopy

Marking Criteria Vomiting Blood	Marks	
	Awarded	Available
Washes hands at the start of the station		1
Introduces themselves – Including First name, last name and role		1
Patient details confirmed: Full name, Age/ D.O.B.		1
Explains purpose of consultation		1
Open question about what brings the patient in today + Clarification of any ambiguity		1
Timeline allows a clear understanding of onset and progression - Onset/ Circumstance - Sudden vs. gradual - Fluctuations - Progression - Past episodes		3
Symptoms elicited are relevant and clearly directed at either arriving at a diagnosis or excluding other plausible diagnoses - Blood o Appearance; Amount - Vomit - Pain - Reflux - Trauma - "RA" – Retching, Alcohol binge		5
Systems queried are relevant to the complaint and adequate questions are asked for each symptom - Gastrointestinal; Constitutional		5
Explores **Ideas, Concerns and Expectations**		3
Elicits relevant **Past Medical History** - Bleeding disorder; PUD or tummy varices; cancer; Liver disease; Recent procedures (Ex. endoscopy); Alcohol-related problems		2
Elicits relevant **Drug History** including **Allergies**		2
Elicits relevant **Family History**		2
Elicits relevant **Social History** – including Smoking/ alcohol/ recreational drugs; **H**ome environment and support; **O**ccupation and impact on life		2
Closes consultation appropriately allowing the patient to ask any questions		1
Presentation: structured, concise		2
Appropriate Differential Diagnosis ± Investigations ± Management Plan		3
Examiner mark – professionalism and rapport		5
Patient mark – professionalism and rapport		5

Consultation	Presentation	Global marks patient	Global marks examiner	Total
30	5	5	5	45

20F presents with blood in vomit

HPC	Noticed blood in vomit. Had been vomiting a lot over the last day – was normal, food and liquid but noticed fresh red blood in the last couple of vomits. Not large amounts – 2 tea spoons perhaps. Had been out for a night on the town yesterday evening and drank a bit much, and thinks that caused the vomiting. Has some abdominal pain, mostly when vomiting but persists a little after – generalised pain, no radiation, tight feeling. No diarrhoea / fevers / travel history / bad food / ill contacts / weight loss / lethargy / night sweats
PMH	Eczema
DH	Emollients
FH	Asthma
SH	Lives with flatmates, university student. Social smoker 5/week, EtOH – at weekends 20 units
ICE	"I'm really scared about the blood, what does it mean?"
Dx	Mallory Weiss Tear
Ix	FBC to ensure stable Hb, none other needed as no red flags
Mx	Reassurance and supportive treatment as needed for vomiting

25M with Haematemesis

HPC	Sudden onset 1-day history of haematemesis. Patient says he has been feeling unwell, vomiting and tired. Complaining of nausea and loss of appetite. He finds it difficult to focus and is less motivated than normally. He describes ongoing central burning abdominal pain, but no chest pain or SOB. Says pain is of sudden onset. Patient says he has had a bad headache and has had diarrhoea. Says he cannot remember parts of the previous night. Has been vomiting 8-10 times over the last day, finds himself retching. Small amounts of blood in spit and vomitus. Fresh, mixed with phlegm and vomitus. Reports no PR bleeding or altered stool colour. No dizziness. Says he went out with his friends the previous night.
PMHx	Nil. Fit and well.
DHx	Nil regular, ibuprofen PRN
FHx	Grandfather diagnosed with oesophageal cancer age 70.
SHx	Works as carpenter. Lives alone. Single. Drinks regularly when out with friends. No smoking. Says he drinks 5 units per day.
ICE	"Doctor, I'm really worried, I don't understand why I'm suddenly vomiting blood. I'm really worried that this is something serious."
Ix	FBC, LFT, coagulation screen, amylase, CRP, CXR, endoscopy
Dx	Mallory-Weiss tears secondary to retching induced by excess alcohol consumption/alcohol associated gastritis.
Tx	Supportive, consider IVI, monitor for acute withdrawal syndrome. Endoscopic injection if severe.

40M with Haematemesis

HPC	Sudden onset large volume haematemesis. He is unable to give precise history of onset. This is the first episode of fresh blooding. He feels very sick and lethargic, tired and his friend told him that "he looks white as a sheet". He feels dizzy and light headed and thinks his heart is racing intermittently. He also feels breathless sweaty, shaky, cold and clammy. He has had previous PR bleeding, diagnosed to be haemorrhoid associated, patient did not attend further follow-up clinic appointments and was subsequently discharged.
PMHx	Chronic pancreatitis, Pancreatic pseudocysts, CKD
DHx	Creon, aspirin PRN, NKDA
SHx	Ex-smoker, drinks 25 units of alcohol/day, used to work as lawyer. Currently unemployed
FHx	Nil relevant
ICE	Patient too unwell to give coherent answers, but visibly distressed.
Ix	ABG, FBC, LFT, coagulation screen, U&E, blood culture, Endoscopy, abdominal x-ray.
Dx	Bleeding oesophageal varices secondary to alcoholic liver disease
Tx	Admit to hospital. IV access and fluid resuscitation, Risk assess (Blatchford score), stop aspirin pre-endoscopy, **Endoscopy + Rockall score calculation**, with varices – sclerotherapy (gastric varices) or banding (oesophageal varices), if failed repeat endoscopy with either Endoscopic balloon insertion (Sengstaken tube) or Trans jugular intrahepatic portosystemic shunting (TIPS) if needed. Blood transfusions. Consider long-term secondary prophylaxis with PO propranolol (C/I asthma) or repeated banding. Alcohol detox regimen according to local protocol (pabrinex/chlordiazepoxide). Alcohol liaison nurse/BIDA.

50F with Haematemesis

HPC	Patient with 3-day history of haematemesis. Small volume, black, coagulated blood intermixed with food. Recurring episodes after meals. Complaining of acute epigastric pain, worse when eating, tends to improve after a while. No fevers. No headaches. No PR bleeding. Reports diarrhoea and says stool has "funny colour" and smells offensive. No coughs, colds or fever. No foreign travel. Says she feels more tired and has trouble falling asleep. Feels sharp pain in abdomen when laying down. Improves when sitting up. Says he has been struggling with back pain for a while following pulling his back doing some DIY, has been self-medicating at home as he is too busy to go and see his GP.
PMHx	Back pain for 10 years, angina, diet controlled T2DM
DHx	Ibuprofen, aspirin, paracetamol, simvastatin
FHx	Nil relevant.
SHx	Works as an accountant for small business. Divorced. No children. Non-smoker. 2 unit per day alcohol consumption.
ICE	"Doctor, I don't understand what is going on. This is really worrying me. You read all these things in the NEWS about cancer and blood, so of course now I'm concerned. And I did a little search on google, and it says that I could have stomach cancer. Do you think that's the case?"
Ix	FBC, U&E, LFT, coagulation screen, PR, Stool sample, erect chest x-ray, abdominal x-ray, Endoscopy.
Dx	Bleeding gastric ulcer
Tx	PPIs, eradication of H. Pylori, Stop NSAIDs

DIARRHOEA
GENERAL FRAMEWORK

"WIPE" – Introduce yourself, whilst gaining consent
- Wash hands
- Introduce self – "Hello, my name is X and I am a medical student"
- Patient details – "Could I ask your full name and age?"
- Explain – "I have been asked to speak with you about what brings you in, would that be alright?"

Open
- I understand you've come in with some diarrhoea. Do you mind telling me about what's been going on?
- Clarify –
  ➤ Have you been more often or is it more liquid?

Timeline
1. When did this start? Anything you think make have triggered it?
2. Did this change in bowels come on suddenly or gradually?
3. Does it come and go or is it there all the time?
4. Has it been getting worse?
5. Have you ever had it before?

Symptoms
- **Stool** – Remember as **"AAFI"**
  ➤ **Amount** - How much?
  ➤ **Appearance** – Consistency? Colour? Content – Blood? Mucus?
  ➤ **Frequency** - How often?
  ➤ **Incomplete emptying** – Do you often feel like you need to go again after having just been to the toilet?

If thinking IBD – ask about back pain/ stiffness; mouth ulcers; anal tags; fever; painful red eye / Spinal cord lesion

Systems
- **Gastrointestinal** – How has your appetite been? Have you had any problems swallowing? Have you been sick at all? ±Blood? Have you had any tummy pain? (Bloating? Wind? – IBS)
- **Genitourinary** – Have you had any problems with the waterworks?
- **Psychiatric** – How has your mood been? Have you been feeling particularly anxious recently?
- **Constitutional** – How has your appetite been? Have you noticed a change in weight? Have you been feeling tired recently? Have you had a fever? Night-sweats? Any joint pain or stiffness?
- **Gynaecological** – Sexually active? Any chance you could be pregnant? LMP?
- **+Food, drink & Exercise** – How is your **diet**? Enough fibre? Water? Do you exercise regularly?
- **+ Travel** – Have you travelled anywhere recently? Ate anything more exotic?

ICE
- You've given me a lot of information, thank you. I'd like to hear a little about what you think could be going on. Do you have any idea?
- Is there anything that's particularly concerning you that you'd like to discuss?
- What exactly are you looking for today, resolution or reassurance?

PMHx
- Do you have any medical conditions?
- Ask a few specific questions to show that you're thinking about different causes
- Specifically, I'd like to ask if you've ever been diagnosed with:
  ➤ Any bowel conditions? Irritable bowels? Cancer?

DHx
- On any medication? Any doses of medication changed?
  - ➤ Specifically ask: Any laxatives? Antibiotics? Indigestion medication?
- Any allergies?

FHx
- Any conditions run in the family? Specifically, I'd like to ask about bowel problems? Colorectal cancer? Something called an autoimmune condition?
- Does anyone in the family also have diarrhoea at the moment?

SHx –
- Smoking/ Alcohol/ Recreational drugs
- Home environment? Support?
- Occupation – impact on life and on occupation?

Summarise and Thank
- I'd just like to summarise back to you to make sure I haven't missed anything
- Is there anything you'd like to talk about that we haven't quite addressed?
- Thank you for talking to me and I wish you all the best

Investigations

Examination	Abdominal exam, thyroid exam (if indicated in history)
Bedside	BP, HR, temperature, weight and BMI.
Bloods	FBC, U&E, CRP, anti-TTG, TFTs, CEA
Imaging	AXR, CT CAP
Special	Colonoscopy, CT CAP, stool MC&S incl. OC&P

Differential Diagnosis

	Diagnosis	Features In History	Features In Investigations	Management
INFECTIVE	**Diverticulitis**	Diarrhoea and LLQ pain, with fevers and rigors. Usually elderly with a history of constipation. Stool may be mixed with blood. Poor diet.	Tender LLQ, no guarding unless complications (perforation / abscess). Raised WCC and CRP.	NBM, IV fluids, ceftriaxone and Metronidazole. Re-introduce low fibre diet then long term for high fibre diet and education.
	Giardia	Diarrhoea >1 week, very flatulent, foul smelling stools, travel to endemic regions (Russia), bloated and generally unwell.	Giardia on stool MC&S including ova, cysts and parasites.	Rehydrate if needed, Metronidazole. May get Malabsorption.
	Gastroenteritis	Sudden onset, diarrhoea and vomiting with urgency, sick contacts or close living quarters (halls / nursing home / recent admission), fever, myalgia, lethargy.	Raised WCC and CRP may be present	Usually viral and self-terminating.
NON-INFECTIVE	**Cancer**	Change in bowel habit (may alternate with constipation), weight loss (quantify!), lethargy, anorexia. RF: FH, previous polyps, smoking	Iron deficiency anaemia, raised WCC/CRP. Obstruction on AXR. CT CAP for staging CT. Colonoscopy for diagnosis (biopsy)	Surgical resection usually. Regular screening colonoscopies.
	IBD	Frequent, intermittent, chronic, loose stools (may be bloody / have mucous), weight loss, anorexia, lethargy. Extra intestinal: eyes, joint pains, skin rashes, perianal abscess	Generalised abdominal tenderness, may have RIF mass (ileocecal) Raised WCC, CRP. Faecal calprotectin raised. AXR may show thumb printing. Colonoscopy for biopsy (?transmural inflammation)	Rehydrate, Immunosuppression (prednisolone, azathioprine / 5- MP, infliximab etc. depending on response)
	IBS	Diarrhoea, no blood, alternating with constipation, cramps and bloating. Discomfort relieved by defecation, worse on eating. No weight loss, anorexia or systemic upset. F > M.	Few findings on examination and investigations – must do to rule out more sinister causes of diarrhoea.	Lifestyle advice, regular meals, fluids. Increase fibre in diet. Medical: for prominent symptom (diarrhoea vs constipation vs cramps)
	Hyperthyroidism	Diarrhoea, heat intolerance, weight loss, increased appetite, tachycardia /palpitations, tremor. Other autoimmune diseases.	Raised T4 and low TSH. Positive findings on examination for hyperthyroid.	"block and replace" therapy with carbimazole and thyroxine if clinically significant.

Also Consider: Laxative abuse and coeliac disease

10M with diarrhoea and vomiting

HPC	Mother reports sudden onset severe diarrhoea and vomiting for 2 days. Reports significant abdominal pain. Fever and headaches. Says he often finds himself having diarrhoea and needing to vomit at the same time. Has been spending the last days in the bathroom. Unable to eat or drink. Feels his mouth is very dry he feels thirsty. Mum found that the heart was beating faster than usual. Her two other children have had similar symptoms and are recovering but they were not as bad as he is. No haemoptysis. No PR bleed. No foreign travel. No confusion or LOC. No seizures. No recent travel. Not confused. Anxious.
PMHx	Nil, fit and healthy
DHx	Paracetamol PRN, nil regular, NKDA
FHx	Nil relevant.
SHx	Lives with parents and grandparents at home. 2 siblings. Parents both work in hospital.
Ix	FBC, LFT, U&E, stool culture
Dx	Viral Gastroenteritis (Norovirus)
Tx	Supportive treatment, IVI fluids

25M with diarrhoea

HPC	2-weeks history of diarrhoea that recently has become bloody, blood mixed in with faeces, some mucus as well. Severe abdominal pain. Low-grade fever. Has noticed weight loss but unable to specify quantity. Patient reports having had similar episodes before, but never with blood in stool. Abdomen feels bloated. Complaining of difficulty in swallowing as he has a sore mouth. No rash, CP, SOB or palpitations, vomiting, nausea joint pain/swelling. Denies unprotected sex/foreign travel or urethral discharge. Reports no IV drug use.
PMHx	Nil
DHx	Paracetamol PRN, NKDA
SHx	Lives alone, occasional alcohol intake, smoking for 10 years; 20 a day.
ICE	"Doctor, I wasn't really worried when it was just the diarrhoea, but now that there's blood in it, I'm getting more worried. What is going on?"
Ix	FBC, U&E, LFT, CRP, Blood cultures, abdomen X-ray, CT abdo pelvis, consider endoscopy
Dx	Crohn's Disease
Tx	No cure, symptom control, anti-inflammatory (5ASAs), steroids, to control inflammatory response, immunosuppression (Azathioprine, ciclosporin, Methotrexate) and biological agents like Infliximab/Adalimumab advise smoking cessation. Surgery is reserved for complications (bowel obstruction)

60F with vomiting and diarrhoea

HPC	Patient with vomiting and diarrhoea for 2 days. Also reports severe abdominal cramps and pain as well as fever. Diarrhoea contains mucus and pus with the faeces. Also contains some fresh blood. Says it all started after she ate at the local organic chicken market. Reports some dizziness, especially when standing for a long time. Feels febrile and sweaty. She reports no visual disturbances, no SOB, no chest pain, no coughs or colds. No foreign travel. Says her faeces are of a marked black-green colour and smell very strongly and badly.
PMHx	Fibroids, COPD
DHx	Paracetamol PRN, inhalers, NKDA
SHx	Ex-smoker of 20 years, quit 5 years ago. Lives with husband. 1 adult child.
FHx	Nil relevant
ICE	"I feel awful doctor, I feel like I have to go to the toilet all the time and it's getting very uncomfortable. What do you think is going on?"
Ix	FBC, U&E, LFT, CRP, stool sample, abdominal x-ray
Dx	Salmonellosis
Tx	Pain relief, fever control, rehydration, supportive treatment, may require admission if dehydrated or AKI. Usually self-limiting in few days.

Marking Criteria Diarrhoea	Marks	
	Awarded	Available
Washes hands at the start of the station		1
Introduces themselves – Including First name, last name and role		1
Patient details confirmed: Full name, Age/ D.O.B.		1
Explains purpose of consultation		1
Open question about what brings the patient in today + Clarification of any ambiguity – More often vs. more liquid		1
Timeline allows a clear understanding of onset and progression - Onset/ Circumstance - Sudden vs. gradual - Fluctuations - Progression - Past episodes		3
Symptoms elicited are relevant and clearly directed at either arriving at a diagnosis or excluding other plausible diagnoses - Amount - Appearance - Frequency - Incomplete emptying		5
Systems queried are relevant to the complaint and adequate questions are asked for each symptom - Gastrointestinal; Genitourinary; Psychiatric; Constitutional; Gynaecological; **Food/ drink/ exercise; Travel**		5
Explores **Ideas, Concerns and Expectations**		3
Elicits relevant **Past Medical History** - Bowel conditions; Irritable bowels; Cancer		2
Elicits relevant **Drug History** including **Allergies**		2
Elicits relevant **Family History**		2
Elicits relevant **Social History** – including Smoking/ alcohol/ recreational drugs; **Home** environment and support; **Occupation** and impact on life		2
Closes consultation appropriately allowing the patient to ask any questions		1
Presentation: structured, concise		2
Appropriate Differential Diagnosis ± Investigations ± Management Plan		3
Examiner mark – professionalism and rapport		5
Patient mark – professionalism and rapport		5

Consultation	Presentation	Global marks patient	Global marks examiner	Total
30	5	5	5	45

CONSTIPATION
GENERAL FRAMEWORK

"WIPE" – Introduce yourself, whilst gaining consent
- Wash hands
- Introduce self – "Hello, my name is X and I am a medical student"
- Patient details – "Could I ask your full name and age?"
- Explain – "I have been asked to speak with you about what brings you in, would that be alright?"

Open
- I understand you've come in with some constipation. Do you mind telling me about what's been going on?
- Clarify –
    - Have you been going less or have you noticed harder stool?

Timeline
1. When did this start? Anything you think make have triggered it?
2. Did this change in bowels come on suddenly or gradually?
3. Does it come and go or is it there all the time?
4. Has it been getting worse?
5. Have you ever had it before?

Symptoms
- **Stool** – Remember as **"AAFI"**
    - **Amount** - How much?
    - **Appearance** – Consistency? Colour? Content – Blood? Mucus?
    - **Frequency** - How often?
    - **Incomplete emptying** – Do you often feel like you need to go again after having just been to the toilet?

Systems
- **Gastrointestinal** – How has your appetite been? Have you had any problems swallowing? Have you been sick at all? ±Blood? Have you had any tummy pain?
- **Genitourinary** – Have you had any problems with the waterworks?
- **Psychiatric** – How has your mood been? Have you been feeling particularly anxious recently?
- **Constitutional** – How has your appetite been? Have you noticed a change in weight? Have you been feeling tired recently? Have you had a fever? Night-sweats?
- **Gynaecological** – Sexually active? Any chance you could be pregnant? LMP?
- **+Food, drink & Exercise** – How is your diet? Do you exercise regularly?
- **+ Travel** – Have you travelled anywhere recently? Ate anything more exotic?

ICE
- You've given me a lot of information, thank you. I'd like to hear a little about what you think could be going on. Do you have any idea?
- Is there anything that's particularly concerning you that you'd like to discuss?
- What exactly are you looking for today, resolution or reassurance?

PMHx
- Do you have any medical conditions?
- Ask a few specific questions to show that you're thinking about different causes
- Specifically, I'd like to ask if you've ever been diagnosed with:
    - Any bowel conditions? Irritable bowels? Cancer? Prior surgery? (Adhesions ⬜ constipation)

DHx
- On any medication? Any doses of medication changed?
  - ➤ Specifically ask: Any painkillers? Calcium channel blockers? Antidepressants (TCAs are anticholinergic)? Iron tablets?
- Any allergies?

FHx
- Any conditions run in the family? Specifically, I'd like to ask about bowel problems? Colorectal cancer? Something called an autoimmune condition?
- Does anyone in the family also have diarrhoea at the moment?

SHx –
- Smoking/ Alcohol/ Recreational drugs
- Home environment? Support?
- Occupation – impact on life and on occupation?

Summarise and Thank
- I'd just like to summarise back to you to make sure I haven't missed anything
- Is there anything you'd like to talk about that we haven't quite addressed?
- Thank you for talking to me and I wish you all the best

Investigations

Examination	Abdominal examination (?masses) including hernia orifices
Bedside	Urinalysis, temperature
Bloods	FBC, U&E, bone profile, TFTs, CEA, iron studies
Imaging	AXR, CT abdomen
Special	Rigid sigmoidoscopy, colonoscopy

Differential Diagnosis

	Diagnosis	Features In History	Features In Investigations	Management
SURGICAL	**Bowel obstruction (ileus, hernia, adhesions, malignancy etc.)**	Nausea and vomiting (feculent in late obstruction) associated with constipation, obstipation, abdominal distension, Abdominal pain. May be ileus after abdominal surgery or obstructing cancer (ask about red flags, B symptoms, previous colonoscopies)	Abdominal distension, generalised tenderness, absent or "tinkling" bowel sounds. AXR: dilated bowel loops, perhaps fluid levels. (Look for perforation: Rigler's sign or air under diaphragm in erect CXR). Gastrograffin follow through may show apple core sign in cancer.	"Drip and suck" – IV fluids, NG tube on free drainage and treat underlying cause of obstruction.
	Cancer	Change in bowel habit (may alternate with diarrhoea), possibly mixed with blood (ranging from fresh to digested), weight loss (quantify!), lethargy, anorexia. RF: FH, previous polyps, smoking	Iron deficiency anaemia, raised WCC/CRP. Obstruction on AXR. CT CAP for staging CT. Colonoscopy for diagnosis (biopsy)	Surgical resection usually; may get adjunct radio- / chemo- therapy. Regular screening colonoscopies.
MEDICAL	**Hypothyoidism**	Reduced frequency of bowels opening, not hard. with weight gain, cold intolerance, lethargy, irregular periods. May have other autoimmune diseases (vitiligo, T1DM) or family history.	Examination: Dry skin, depressed reflexes, goitre. No PR findings. Bloods: Raised TSH, low T4.	Thyroxine, titrated to TFTs. Symptomatic relief with laxatives if needed.
	Medication	History of constipation worsening after starting new meds / post op (opioids for analgesia) with no laxatives. May also be anti-cholinergic (anti-psychotics)	Review of medications Normal bloods	Laxatives whilst on constipating medications. Advice re: fibre and fluid in diet.
	IBS	Constipation, no blood, alternating with diarrhoea, cramps and bloating. Discomfort relieved by defecation, worse on eating. No weight loss, anorexia or systemic upset. F > M.	Few findings on examination and investigations – must do to rule out more sinister causes of diarrhoea.	Lifestyle advice, regular meals, fluids. Increase fibre in diet. Medical: for prominent symptom (diarrhoea vs constipation vs cramps)
	Other Common Causes: Poor Diet, poor hydration and pain on defecation			

45F with constipation

HPC	Patient complaining of constipation for 1 week. Had elective knee replacement 9 days ago. Last BO 8 days ago. Feels sore tummy on left side and feel bloated. No urinary incontinence, No dysuria. No fever. He has never been troubled with constipation. No nausea, vomiting, night sweats, fever or weight loss. Denies any pain during defecation or blood in stool. He is not eating very well. Reduced mobility post-op due to concerns about bleeding. Also says he is afraid that moving will hurt. Very anxious.
PMHx	Fibromyalgia
DHx	Codeine, Tramadol, Oromorph PRN for fibromyalgia, doses increased post op.
FHx	Nil.
SHx	Lives with husband, no children. Non-smoker. Takes 2 units of alcohol/per day, 6 on weekend. Works in in car company.
ICE	"Doctor, this is madness. I'm already in pain with my fibromyalgia; I can't deal with the pain of my knee and from not being able to open my bowels. I sit on the toilet, but nothing happens."
Ix	FBC, U&E, CRP, LFT, wound check, PR, abdominal x-ray
Dx	Opiate induced constipation.
Tx	Enema/suppository to alleviate constipation, long term laxatives whilst on opiates.

35F with fevers and constipation

HPC	Patient with 2-weeks history of gradually increasing fever as well as constipation and abdominal pain. Complaining of headaches and loss of appetite. Patient also reports some gradually worsening weakness and general malaise and feels exhausted. Foreign travel to India 2 weeks ago. Patient also reports a rash of on her chest and abdomen. She also complaints of distended abdomen, no nausea, vomiting but feels her appetite is reduced. No palpitations or dizziness. No cough or colds. No haemoptysis. No medication changes. She took her malaria prophylaxis religiously and was not bitten by mosquitoes. No dysuria/haematuria but feels achy all over. She denies any headache.
PMHx	Nil. Normally fit and well.
DHx	NKDA, paracetamol for pain, multivitamin.
SHx	Works in a sandwich factory, married. 2 Children. Non-smoker, drinks very occasionally.
FHx	Nil relevant
ICE	"Doctor, I'm supposed to go to work, but I just can't do it. How long will this will take?"
Ix	FBC, CRP, Blood cultures, stool sample/culture, CXR, Abdo-X-ray
Dx	Typhoid fever
Tx	Ciprofloxacin or Ceftriaxone

82F with constipation

HPC	2-weeks history of constipation. Patient normally in residential home. Reported to be more confused and irritable. Patient reports headaches and difficulty in concentrating. She also complains of her arthritis being more painful than usually. Reports nausea and vomiting as well as abdominal pain. Reports being thirstier than usual. Denies any increased frequency of micturition or dysuria. Does not wake up at night to pass urine, no fever. Unsure of weight loss as she has not checked her weight recently. No SOB, CP or palpitations. No dizziness. No foreign travel.
PMHx	Breast cancer diagnosed 16 years ago, Dementia. T2DM with CKD stage 5 (refused dialysis).
DHx	Metformin, gliclazide, insulin, Calcichew D3 forte. NKDA
FHx	Mother diagnosed with bowel cancer age 70
SHx	Lives in residential home. Non-smoker. No alcohol. Normally independent in most activities of daily living.
ICE	"Doctor, my head hurts and I'm so much twitchier all the time. I can't get my legs to calm down."
Ix	FBC, U&E, CRP, LFT, Bone profile, Vit D, PTH, urine calcium, AXR, renal USG, DEXA scan, CT chest abdo pelvis
Dx	Hypercalcaemia due to secondary hyperparathyroidism as a result of end stage renal disease
Tx	IVI to lower plasma calcium levels and increase excretion, Furosemide, Bisphosphonates, Stope Calcichew D3 forte

Marking Criteria Constipation	Marks	
	Awarded	Available
Washes hands at the start of the station		1
Introduces themselves – Including First name, last name and role		1
Patient details confirmed: Full name, Age/ D.O.B.		1
Explains purpose of consultation		1
Open question about what brings the patient in today + Clarification of any ambiguity –Less often vs. harder stool		1
Timeline allows a clear understanding of onset and progression - Onset/ Circumstance - Sudden vs. gradual - Fluctuations - Progression - Past episodes		3
Symptoms elicited are relevant and clearly directed at either arriving at a diagnosis or excluding other plausible diagnoses - Amount - Appearance - Frequency - Incomplete emptying		5
Systems queried are relevant to the complaint and adequate questions are asked for each symptom - Gastrointestinal; Genitourinary; Psychiatric; Constitutional; Gynaecological; **Food/ drink/ exercise**; **Travel**		5
Explores **Ideas, Concerns and Expectations**		3
Elicits relevant **Past Medical History** - Bowel conditions; Irritable bowels; Cancer		2
Elicits relevant **Drug History** including **Allergies**		2
Elicits relevant **Family History**		2
Elicits relevant **Social History** – including **S**moking/ alcohol/ recreational drugs; **H**ome environment and support; **O**ccupation and impact on life		2
Closes consultation appropriately allowing the patient to ask any questions		1
Presentation: structured, concise		2
Appropriate Differential Diagnosis ± Investigations ± Management Plan		3
Examiner mark – professionalism and rapport		5
Patient mark – professionalism and rapport		5

Consultation	Presentation	Global marks patient	Global marks examiner	Total
30	5	5	5	45

RECTAL BLEED
GENERAL FRAMEWORK

"WIPE" – Introduce yourself, whilst gaining consent
- Wash hands
- Introduce self – "Hello, my name is X and I am a medical student"
- Patient details – "Could I ask your full name and age?"
- Explain – I have been asked to speak with you about what brings you in, would that be alright?

Open
- Open – I understand you've recently noticed some blood in stool, which must have been very distressing. Can you tell me about that?
- Clarify – Can I just clarify where you noticed the blood? Was it on the paper/ pan or was mixed in with the stool? Definitely from your back passage or could be menstruation/ in urine?

Timeline
1. When did you first notice the bleeding? Did anything happen around then?
2. Did it come on suddenly or gradually?
3. Does the bleeding come and go or is it always there?
4. Has it been getting worse?
5. Have you had bleeding like this before?

Symptoms
- Blood
  - **Colour** – Is the blood bright red or dark and "tar-like"?
  - **Amount** – How much blood would you say there is? Splatters; spoonfuls; cupfuls?
- Stool – **"AAFI"**
  - **Amount** - How much?
  - **Appearance** – Consistency? Colour? Content – Blood? Mucus?
  - **Frequency** - How often?
  - **Incomplete emptying** – Do you often feel like you need to go again after having just been to the toilet?
- Others –
  - **Pain** – Do you have any pain on passing stool?
  - **Itchiness** – Do you have any itchiness in your back passage?
  - **Lumps** – Have you noticed any lumps in your back passage?

Systems
- **Gastrointestinal** – How has your appetite been? Have you had any problems swallowing? Have you been sick at all? ±Blood? Have you had any tummy pain? **How have your bowel movements been, other than the blood?**
- **Constitutional** – How has your appetite been? Have you noticed a change in weight? Have you been feeling tired recently? Have you had a fever? Night-sweats?
- **+Food, drink & Exercise** – How is your diet? Do you exercise regularly?
- **+ Travel** – Have you travelled anywhere recently? Ate anything more exotic?

ICE
- You've given me a lot of information, thank you. I'd like to hear a little about what you think could be going on. Do you have any idea?
- Is there anything that's particularly concerning you that you'd like to discuss?
- What exactly are you looking for today, resolution or reassurance?

PMHx
- Do you have any medical conditions?
- Ask a few specific questions to show that you're thinking about different causes
- Specifically, I'd like to ask if you've ever been diagnosed with: "**AABBCP**"
  > Anal fissures? Anal prolapse? Bleeding disorders? Bowel problems (Inflammatory bowel

DHx
- On any medication? Any doses of medication changed?
  > Specifically ask: Any laxatives? Blood thinning medication?
- Any allergies?

FHx
- Any conditions run in the family? Specifically, I'd like to ask about bowel problems? Colorectal cancer? Bleeding disorders?
- Has anyone in the family passed blood in their stool like this before?

SHx
- Smoking/ Alcohol/ Recreational drugs
- Home environment? Support?
- Occupation – impact on life and on occupation?

Summarise and Thank
- I'd just like to summarise back to you to make sure I haven't missed anything
- Is there anything you'd like to talk about that we haven't quite addressed?
- Thank you for talking to me and I wish you all the best

Investigations

Examination	Abdominal examination (?CLD signs), digital rectal examination
Bedside	Urinalysis, temperature
Bloods	FBC, clotting, U&E, CEA, LFTs, amylase, lactate, CRP
Imaging	AXR, CT abdomen
Special	Proctoscopy, colonoscopy, stool MC&S incl. OC&P, faecal calprotectin

Top Tip! **When should you refer someone with PR Bleeding?**
This depends on if they have high risk features e.g. anorexia, change in bowel habit, lethargy
  > Any Age + high risk features → Refer to colorectal clinic
  > Above 40 + No high risk features → Flexible Sigmoidoscopy
  > Below 40 + No high risk features → Conservative Management

Differential Diagnosis

	Diagnosis	Features In History	Features In Investigations	Management
STRUCTURAL	Cancer	PR blood (ranging from fresh → melena) associated with change in bowel habit, weight loss (quantify!), lethargy, anorexia. RF: FH, previous polyps, smoking	DRE: may feel rectal mass. Bloods: Iron deficiency anaemia, raised CEA, WCC/CRP. Obstruction on AXR. CT CAP for staging CT. Colonoscopy for diagnosis (biopsy)	Surgical resection usually; may get adjunct radio- / chemo- therapy. Regular screening colonoscopies.
	Haemorrhoids	Painless fresh red blood usually on top of stool and on toilet paper. May feel lump (does it go back inside? Can you push it back?). Are they tender (thrombosed)? RF: History of constipation	DRE: external haemorrhoids visible, or internal haemorrhoids palpable.	Depends on grade and symptoms. Thrombosed haemorrhoids need surgical intervention if within 48 hours. Advice to keep stools soft (diet, hydration), simple analgesia, topical steroids.
	Anal Fissure	Fresh red blood on toilet paper, fleeting, severe, sharp pain on defecation. Very tender. May be associated with constipation (hard stool as cause of fissure and due to trying to avoid pain from fissure).	DRE: may see fissure, internal examination in very uncomfortable for patient. No masses.	Advice to keep stools soft (diet, hydration), simple analgesia, warm baths, GTN ointment if no improvement.
NON - STRUCTURAL	Upper GI bleed (above ligament of Treitz)	Melena (black, sticky, foul smelling stool), associated with epigastric discomfort, may have haematemesis. Ass. with history of oesophageal varices and peptic ulcer disease.	Exam: signs of chronic liver disease. DRE: no masses or fresh blood, melena. Bloods: low Hb, high urea (protein meal), deranged LFTs.	Urgent assessment of haemodynamic stability, admit → OGD. Calculate Blatchford and Rockall scores.
	Inflammatory Bowel Disease (UC > Crohn's)	Frequent, intermittent, chronic, bloody/mucous loose stools, weight loss, anorexia, lethargy. Extra intestinal: eyes, joint pains, skin rashes, perianal abscess.	Generalised abdominal tenderness, may have RIF mass (ileocecal) Raised WCC, CRP. Faecal calprotectin raised. AXR may show thumb printing. Colonoscopy for biopsy (?transmural inflammation)	Rehydrate, Immunosuppression (prednisolone, azathioprine / 5-MP, infliximab etc. depending on response) to induce remission in acute flare.

Also consider: diverticulitis and haemorrhagic gastroenteritis (Shigella, Campylobacter, Salmonella, Yersinia, E.coli) if infective symptoms present. Rarely, clotting disorders may present with PR bleed.

Marking Criteria Rectal Bleed	Marks	
	Awarded	Available
Washes hands at the start of the station		1
Introduces themselves – Including First name, last name and role		1
Patient details confirmed: Full name, Age/ D.O.B.		1
Explains purpose of consultation		1
Open question about what brings the patient in today + Clarification of any ambiguity – Blood on paper? Pan? Mixed with stool?		1
Timeline allows a clear understanding of onset and progression - Onset/ Circumstance - Sudden vs. gradual - Fluctuations - Progression - Past episodes		3

Symptoms elicited are relevant and clearly directed at either arriving at a diagnosis or excluding other plausible diagnoses
- Blood
   o Colour
   o Amount
- Stool
   o Amount
   o Appearance
   o Frequency
   o Incomplete emptying
- Others
   o Pain
   o Itchiness
   o Lumps
		5

Systems queried are relevant to the complaint and adequate questions are asked for each symptom - Gastrointestinal; Constitutional; **Food/ drink/ exercise**; **Travel**		5
Explores **Ideas, Concerns and Expectations**		3
Elicits relevant **Past Medical History** - Bowel conditions; Irritable bowels; Cancer		2
Elicits relevant **Drug History** including **Allergies**		2
Elicits relevant **Family History**		2
Elicits relevant **Social History** – including Smoking/ alcohol/ recreational drugs; Home environment and support; **O**ccupation and impact on life		2
Closes consultation appropriately allowing the patient to ask any questions		1
Presentation: structured, concise		2
Appropriate Differential Diagnosis ± Investigations ± Management Plan		3
Examiner mark – professionalism and rapport		5
Patient mark – professionalism and rapport		5

Consultation	Presentation	Global marks patient	Global marks examiner	Total
30	5	5	5	45

85F with 5 weeks of PR bleed.

HPC	Patient complaining of 5 weeks of PR bleeding. Says blood is mixed in with stool. She also describes that she is passing stool more often and that it is looser. She has been losing weight for recently and has dropped 3 dress sizes. Not actively trying to lose weight. Also describes nausea and vomiting as well as increased fatigue. Sleeps more than usually but has to wake up at night as feels hot and sweaty. No fever, SOB, cough, CP, no infective symptoms.
PMHx	HTN, Crohn's
DHx	Aspirin, bisoprolol, azathioprine, NKDA
FHx	Mother also had Crohn's, nil other.
SHx	Ex-Smoker, quit 20 years ago due to Crohn's, drinks 2 units of alcohol per day, Lives alone, widow
ICE	"Doctor, I'm worried. I'm not young anymore - Do you reckon it is something bad?"
Ix	FBC, iron studies, CRP, LFT, U&E, faecal calprotectin, PR, Colonoscopy, CT abdomen
Dx	Bowel Cancer
Tx	Refer to Specialist MDT for consideration of surgery chemo/radiotherapy. Involve palliative team and McMillan nurses if appropriate

50M with 4 day history of PR bleeding

HPC	4 day history of PR bleeding. Fresh blood when wiping. On paper after opening bowels. Not mixed in with stool, on top of stool and in bowl. Thinks it is large amounts as the water is very red. Usually constipated which is worse in the last week. Increased strain to pass faeces. Painful and itchy rectum. Especially when sitting for long time. Painful when opening bowels. Says he avoids vegetables as he doesn't like the taste and they make him feel bloated. Diet mainly consists of processed food as he travels a lot. Reports no abdominal pain. No systemic symptoms of infection. No nausea, no vomiting, no CP, no SOB
PMHx	HTN, T2DM.
DHx	Metformin, Ramipril, NKDA
SHx	Pub owner, Married. Drinks up to 10 units per day, sometimes more. Non-smoker. Obese.
FHx	Father diagnosed with bowel cancer age 50.
ICE	"I'm worried that I have cancer- my dad had blood in his faeces before he was diagnosed as well."
Ix	FBC, U&E, LFT, Vitamin B and folate, iron studies, consider colonoscopy or CT abdo-pelvis.
Dx	Haemorrhoids
Tx	Conservative management with increased fibre and water intake, topical treatment. Surgery if very troublesome or prolapsing.

17F with PR bleeding and diarrhoea

HPC	Reports 3-months history of diarrhoea and some abdominal pain. Recently blood in stool. Blood mixed with stool. Progressively worsening symptoms. Had episodes of long term diarrhoea in the past, but usually self-resolve. Reports low grade fever and weight loss (unable to quantify) and generally finds it difficult to gain weight. Complaining of sore knees, hips and elbows. Symptoms are particularly worse around her exam times. No lumps and bumps. No night sweats. Reports no SOB, CP or dizziness. No vomiting. No nausea. No Dysuria. Period regular.
PMHx	Menarche age 14, nil otherwise
DHx	Paracetamol for pain PRN, oral contraceptive pill, NKDA
SHx	Non-smoker, does not drink, single, no IVDU or other drug use
FHx	Nil relevant
ICE	"Doctor, I'm so embarrassed by this. I'm constantly running to the toilet because I have diarrhoea and now there's also blood in here and it worries me. I'm tired all the time and getting afraid of leaving the house because I don't want to use my friend's toilets."
Ix	FBC, Vitamin B, folate, faecal calprotectin, LFTs, Endoscopy, Sigmoidoscopy/colonoscopy, AXR
Dx	Ulcerative colitis
Tx	Symptom control, anti-inflammatory (5ASAs), steroids, immunosuppression (Azathioprine, ciclosporin, Methotrexate) and biological agents like Infliximab/Adalimumab. Advise smoking cessation. Surgery is if toxic megacolon or refractory to treatment.

GENITOURINARY HISTORIES

DYSURIA
"WOCC SOCRATES"

"**W**IPE" – Introduce yourself, whilst gaining consent
- Wash hands
- Introduce self – "Hello, my name is X and I am a medical student"
- Patient details – "Could I ask your full name and age?"
- Explain – "I have been asked to speak with you about what brings you in, would that be alright?"

Open
- I understand you've had some pain on passing urine, would you mind telling me more about that?
- **C**larification – Is the pain only when you pass urine or other times also?
- **C**onsider pain relief – You seem to be in a lot of pain. Have you been offered pain relief?

Site
- Where exactly do you feel this pain?

Onset
1. When did the pain start? Did anything happen around then?
2. Did the pain come on suddenly or gradually?
3. Does the pain come and go or is it there every time you urinate?
4. Has the pain been getting worse?
5. Have you ever had pain like this before?

Character
- Can you describe the pain for me? Dull ache/ Stinging, Sharp/ Colicky, Cyclical

Radiation
- Does the pain move anywhere?
- Does it move towards your groin? Towards your back?

Timing – This has been done.

Exacerbating/ relieving factors
- Anything make the pain better or worse?

Severity
- How bad is the pain on a scale of 1 to 10?

PMHx
- Do you have any medical conditions?
- Ask a few specific questions to show that you're thinking about different causes
- Specifically, I'd like to ask if you've ever been diagnosed with:
  - ➤ Urinary tract infections? Prostate problems? Kidney problems? Kidney stones? Sexually transmitted infections? Any recent procedures (cystoscopy, renal surgery, etc.)?

Associated
- **Symptoms "Urine + DRIL"**
  - ➢ **Urine**
    - o Have you been passing **more/less** urine than usual?
    - o Have you noticed any change the **smell** of the urine?
    - o **Colour** of the urine?
    - o Have you seen any **blood** in the urine? How much? How often?
    - o Have you noticed any **foaminess** or **sediment**?
  - ➢ **Discharge** – Have you noticed any discharge from your penis/ vagina?
  - ➢ **Rashes** – Have you noticed any rashes or blisters in your penis/ vagina?
  - ➢ **Illness** – Have you been ill recently?
  - ➢ **Lower Urinary Tract Symptoms**
    - ▪ Do you struggle to initiate the stream of urine? Once you begin urinating, is it a continuous flow? Do you experience any dribbling of urine at the end? Do you ever find that you want to go again after you've just been?

- **Systems**
  - ➢ **Genitourinary** – Other than the pain, how have the waterworks been? Have you been passing urine more/ less often? Have you experienced any incontinence? Retention? Urgency?
  - ➢ **Sexual** – Have you had any unprotected sexual intercourse recently?
  - ➢ **Gynaecological** – How have your period been? Related to periods at all?
  - ➢ **Constitutional** – How has your appetite been? Have you noticed a change in weight? Have you been feeling tired recently? Have you had a fever? Night-sweats?

ICE
- You've given me a lot of information, thank you. I'd like to hear a little about what you think could be going on. Do you have any idea?
- Is there anything that's particularly concerning you that you'd like to discuss?
- What exactly are you looking for today, resolution or reassurance?

DHx
- On any medication? Any doses of medication changed?
  - ➢ Specifically ask: Diuretics (ACE-i)? Long-term antibiotics?
- Any allergies?

FHx
- Any conditions run in the family? Specifically, I'd like to ask about Kidney or bladder problems? Both parents alive and well?
- Has anyone in the family ever had symptoms similar to the ones you're experiencing?

SHx –
- Smoking/ Alcohol/ Recreational drugs
- Home environment? Support?
- Occupation – impact on life and on occupation?

Summarise and Thank
- – I'd just like to summarise back to you to make sure I haven't missed anything
- – Is there anything you'd like to talk about that we haven't quite addressed?
- – Thank you for talking to me and I wish you all the best

Differential Diagnosis

Diagnosis	Features In History	Features In Investigations	Management
UTI	Dysuria associated with urinary frequency, fevers, rigors, suprapubic pain. Urine may appear cloudy / bloody and be odorous. Female, recent catheterisation, elderly are risk factors	Exam: suprapubic tenderness, pyrexia. Bedside: urine positive for leucocytes and nitrites. Bloods: raised WCC, CRP	Antibiotics – trimethoprim 3 days or nitrofurantoin for 5 days.
STI	Dysuria associated with urethral discharge. History of risky sexual activity (multiple partners, no barrier contraception, previous STIs). May have genital rash / systemic symptoms.	Exam: urethral discharge. Swabs positive for gonorrhoea / chlamydia most commonly.	Empirical Antibiotics. For Chlamydia, 1g azithromycin stat (and ceftriaxone if gonococcal), patient education and contact tracing.

Also consider: Endometriosis

Investigations

Examination	Abdominal examination, genito-urinary examination incl. swabs
Bedside	Swabs, temperature, urine dip
Bloods	FBC, U&E (renal impairment)
Imaging	Consider USS KUB incl. Doppler if renal impairment
Special	First pass urine for NAAT, urine MC&S. GUM clinic management of STI.

20M with 1 week history of dysuria

HPC	Patient with 1-week history of dysuria. Sudden onset. Never had this before. Reports painful ulcerative lesions on penis. He has also noticed a rash on his penis but no discharge. Patient admits to unprotected sex 1-week prior to onset of symptoms. Not regular partner. Reports penis feels sore and more sensitive than usually. No abdominal pain, bowel habits unchanged, no haematuria, not systemically unwell. No fever. Denies joint pain or swellings. No foreign travel. Never left UK. Bowels unchanged. His weight has not changed. Has not noticed any lumps.
PMHx	Nil.
DHx	NKDA, nil regular, paracetamol for pain, tried antiseptic cream and disinfectant spray on genitals.
FHx	Nil relevant
SHx	Long term girlfriend. Soldier. Smokes 10 per day. Social alcohol.
ICE	"Doctor, do you think this could be because I slept with that other girl? Do you think it is contagious? Will I have to tell my girlfriend? I don't want her to know that I slept with that other girl. I'm so ashamed! I got drunk and lost control."
Ix	FBC, U&E, LFT, CRP, swab of ulcers, blood culture
Dx	Herpes simplex infection
Tx	Aciclovir, sexual advice, will need to abstain from sex until healed.

25F with 3 days of dysuria

HPC	Patient with 3-days history of dysuria and increased frequency. Has noticed that her urine smells bad and is frothy. Reports no vaginal discharge and no incontinence. Feeling febrile and on checking her temperature it was 38°C. She feels chilly and shaky at times. Has had this few times before. After her recent GP appointment, she remains very worried as she was told that her diabetes is not so good and is worried about losing her eye sight. Feels nauseous but has been able to eat and drink, denies chest pain, SOB, cough. Reports no flank pain, but some mild abdominal discomfort.
PMHx	T1DM for last 6 years, Fit and well, no other medical or surgical history.
DHx	Paracetamol for pain, oral contraceptive pill, insulin. NKDA
FMHx	Nil relevant
SHx	New boyfriend, Student. Drinks socially, 4 units per day on the weekend, nil during week. No Smoking. No drug use.
ICE	"Doctor, is this going to take long to resolve? It's just so uncomfortable."
Ix	FBC, U&E, Urine dip (MSU and cultures), Blood culture
Dx	Lower UTI
Tx	Treat empirically with Nitrofurantoin for 3 days, if symptoms don't improve, switch to trimethoprim. Both oral. Follow local antibiotic policy. Diabetes control, DSN input.

25F with cyclical dysuria over past 12 months

HPC	Patient complaining of cyclical dysuria over the past 12 months after giving birth to her first child. No fever, no discharge, incontinence, rash, joint pain or swelling. She has received antibiotics a few times for similar symptoms without benefit. She feels her dysuria is associated with her menstrual cycle. She also says that she gets cyclical severe abdominal pain associated with her menstrual cycle. Denies bowel changes, used to be on the mirena coil for years prior to becoming pregnant. She finds it little embarrassing as she has lot of pain during intercourse. She had difficulty in getting pregnant initially. Patient reports no haematuria, no PV bleed, no infective symptoms.
PMHx	1 Child, normal PV delivery. Nil other.
DHx	NKDA, Nil regular.
SHx	Lives with husband, no other sexual partners, works as hair dresser, part-time. Social alcohol use, 5 cigarettes per day.
FHx	Dad had lung cancer age 70
ICE	"I've been having stomach cramps for years when I have my period - I can deal with that, but pain on peeing is new, and that is a lot more of a problem. Is there anything you can do to help, doctor?"
Ix	FBC, CRP, U&E, PV examination, urine (MSU/culture), cystoscopy, bimanual, USS pelvis
Dx	Dysuria secondary to endometriosis.
Tx	Progesterone therapy, hormone contraception therapy, danazol/gestrinone

Marking Criteria DYSURIA	Marks	
	Awarded	Available
Washed hands at the start of the station		1
Introduced themselves – Including First name, last name and role		1
Patient details confirmed: Full name, Age/ D.O.B.		1
Explained purpose of consultation		1
Open question about what brings the patient in today + Clarification of any ambiguity		1
Site – Enquires about exact location of pain		1
Onset (Timeline) – Asks questions to provide a clear understanding of onset and progression - Onset/ Circumstance - Sudden vs. gradual - Fluctuations - Progression - Past episodes		3
Character - Obtains an accurate description of the pain (Ex. Stab, ache, colic, etc.)		1
Radiation - Asks about the pain moving anywhere else (Ex. towards groin, back, etc.)		1

Associated symptoms
■ **Symptoms** elicited are relevant and clearly directed at either arriving at a diagnosis or excluding other plausible diagnoses
- Urine
  o Amount; Smell; Colour; Blood; Foaminess/ sediment
- DRIL
  o Discharge
  o Rashes
  o Illness
  o LUTS
■ **Systems** queried are relevant to the complaint and adequate questions are asked for each symptom
- Genitourinary; Gynaecological; Sexual; Constitutional
		6

Timing - This has been done		0
Exacerbation/ Relief - Clearly asks if the patient has noticed any relieving/ exacerbating factors, providing appropriate examples if prompted		1
Severity - Subjective quantitative assessment of pain severity		1
Explores **Ideas, Concerns and Expectations**		3
Elicits relevant **Past Medical History** - Urinary tract infections; Prostate problems; Kidney problems; Kidney stones; STIs; Recent procedures (cystoscopy, renal surgery, etc.)		2
Elicits relevant **Drug History** including **Allergies**		2
Elicits relevant **Family History**		2
Elicits relevant **Social History** – including Smoking/ alcohol/ recreational drugs; Home environment and support; Occupation and impact on life		2
Closes consultation appropriately allowing the patient to ask any questions		1
Presentation: structured, concise		2
Appropriate Differential Diagnosis ± Investigations ± Management Plan		3
Examiner mark – professionalism and rapport		5
Patient mark – professionalism and rapport		5

Consultation	Presentation	Global marks patient	Global marks examiner	Total
30	5	5	5	45

INCONTINENCE & URGENCY
GENERAL FRAMEWORK

"WIPE" – Introduce yourself, whilst gaining consent
- Wash hands
- Introduce self – "Hello, my name is X and I am a medical student"
- Patient details – "Could I ask your full name and age?"
- Explain – "I have been asked to speak with you about what brings you in, would that be alright?"

Open
- I understand you've been experiencing some incontinence/ urgency recently, can you tell me more about what's been going on?
- Clarify -

Timeline
1. When did this start? Did anything happen then?
2. Was it something that started suddenly or that you gradually noticed?
3. Does it come and go on occasion or does it happen regularly?
4. Has it been getting worse?
5. Have you ever had anything like this before?

Symptoms
- **Incontinence**
  - ➤ **Frequency** – How often are you incontinent of urine?
  - ➤ **Amount** – How much do you usually leak when you are incontinent?
  - ➤ **Stress/Urgency** – Does it happen when you strain, cough, laugh OR is it more associated with a sudden urge to go?
  - ➤ **Stool** – Are you ever incontinent of stool?
- **Urine**
  - ➤ Have you been passing more/less urine than usual?
  - ➤ Have you noticed any change in the smell of the urine?
  - ➤ What about the colour of the urine?
  - ➤ Have you seen any blood in your urine? How much? How often?
  - ➤ Have you noticed any foaminess or sediment?
- **Lower Urinary Tract Symptoms**
  - ➤ Do you struggle to initiate the stream of urine? Once you begin urinating, is it a continuous flow? Do you experience any dribbling of urine at the end? Do you ever find that you want to go again after you've just been?

Systems
- **Neurological** – Have you had a headache? Noticed a change in any of your senses? And what about any weakness or altered sensation?
- **Genitourinary** –How have the waterworks been? Have you had any pain on passing urine? Have you been passing urine more/ less often?
- **Anxiety** – Would you consider yourself an anxious person? Do you think this could be related to anxiety at all?
- **Sexual** – Have you had any unprotected sexual intercourse recently?
- **Constitutional** – How has your appetite been? Have you noticed a change in weight? Have you been feeling tired recently? Have you had a fever? Night-sweats?

ICE
- You've given me a lot of information, thank you. I'd like to hear a little about what you think could be going on. Do you have any idea?
- Is there anything that's particularly concerning you that you'd like to discuss?
- What exactly are you looking for today, resolution or reassurance?

PMHx
- Do you have any medical conditions?
- Ask a few specific questions to show that you're thinking about different causes
- Specifically, I'd like to ask if you've ever been diagnosed with:
  - Urinary tract infections? Prostate problems? A stroke? A neurological problem? Diabetes mellitus? Diabetes insipidus? Any recent procedures or childbirth? Menopause?

DHx
- On any medication? Any doses of medication changed?
  - Specifically ask: Any BP medication?
- Any allergies?

FHx
- Any conditions run in the family? Specifically, I'd like to ask about urinary problems? Neurological problems?
- Has anyone in the family ever had symptoms similar to the ones you're experiencing?

SHx –
- Smoking/ Alcohol/ Recreational drugs
- Home environment? Support?
- Occupation – impact on life and on occupation?

Summarise and Thank
- I'd just like to summarise back to you to make sure I haven't missed anything
- Is there anything you'd like to talk about that we haven't quite addressed?
- Thank you for talking to me and I wish you all the best

Investigations	
Examination	Abdominal exam ± PV / DRE
Bedside	Urine dip, temperature, blood glucose, BP, HR
Bloods	U&E, FBC, CRP, HbA1c
Imaging	Bladder scan, USS KUB
Special	Urodynamic studies, urine MC&S, urine protein:creatinine ratio

Top Tip! Urinary Tract Infection (UTI) is a broad term that encompasses infections in any part of the urinary tract. Upper UTIs (pyelonephritis) will present with fever and loin pain in addition to the features normally associated with lower UTIs (uretheritis, cystitis) e.g. frequency, dysuria, haematuria.

Differential Diagnosis

	Diagnosis	Features In History	Features In Investigations	Management
ACUTE	**UTI**	Dysuria, frequency, small amounts of urine. Associated with fevers, myalgia, feeling unwell.	Exam: May have tender epigastrium, fever, foul smelling urine. Urine dip: positive leucocytes and nitrites. Bloods: raised WCC and CRP	Antibiotics – trimethoprim or nitrofurantoin. Also assess features of sepsis and need for fluid resuscitation.
	Neurogenic e.g. Stroke / MS / PD	Urgency to go is main problem, cannot hold urine. Complicated by cognitive impairment in elderly.	Signs of underlying cause. Urine dip: NAD	Underlying cause.
CHRONIC	**Diabetes Mellitus**	Polyuria, polydipsia, tiredness, weight loss, FH of DM, personal history of other autoimmune diseases.	Exam: may seem tired, dehydrated. Urine dip: glucose. Bloods: high glucose, HbA1c.	Rehydration, check for DKA and treat if present as emergency. Endocrinology referral.
	Stress Incontinence	Small amounts of urine leak on coughing / sneezing / laughing /heavy lifting. Usually able to control, no urgency, normal bowel habit. RF: female, multiple births, large babies, episiotomies, old age, hysterectomy	Bladder chart for 3 days – no features of frequency or urgency. Negative urine dip. Urodynamic studies (on failure of conservative management) to confirm diagnosis.	Pelvic floor exercises, may try oxybutynin.
	Urge Incontinence	Urgency to pass urine suddenly, unable to get to toilet in time, small volume of urine. RFs: UTI, MS, Parkinson's, elderly, obesity, prostatic enlargement	Exam: sensitive suprapubically. Urine: may show leucocytes and nitrites if UTI Bladder diary may help	Bladder training. Oxybutinin / tolterodine.
	BPH	Small amounts of urine leak, increased frequency and urgency but small amounts of urine with difficulty initiating and completing, terminal dribbling. (essentially overflow incontinency)	Enlarged prostate on DRE (smooth in BPH, nodular / asymmetrical in cancer)	BPH medication when cancer excluded – tamsulosin, finasteride.

Also consider: Iatrogenic e.g. post-Prostatectomy and Post-partum

Marking Criteria Incontinence/ Urgency	Marks	
	Awarded	Available
Washes hands at the start of the station		1
Introduces themselves – Including First name, last name and role		1
Patient details confirmed: Full name, Age/ D.O.B.		1
Explains purpose of consultation		1
Open question about what brings the patient in today + Clarification of any ambiguity		1
Timeline allows a clear understanding of onset and progression - Onset/ Circumstance - Sudden vs. gradual - Fluctuations - Progression - Past episodes		3

Symptoms elicited are relevant and clearly directed at either arriving at a diagnosis or excluding other plausible diagnoses
 - Incontinence
   o Frequency; Amount; Stress vs Urgency; Stool
 - Urine
   o Amount; Smell; Appearance; Blood; Foaminess/ sediment
 - LUTS
		5

Systems queried are relevant to the complaint and adequate questions are asked for each symptom - Neurological; Genitourinary; Anxiety; Sexual; Constitutional		5
Explores **Ideas, Concerns and Expectations**		3
Elicits relevant **Past Medical History** - UTIs; Prostate problems; Past stroke; Neurological problem; DM; DI; Recent procedures or childbirth; Menopause		2
Elicits relevant **Drug History** including **Allergies**		2
Elicits relevant **Family History**		2
Elicits relevant **Social History** – including Smoking/ alcohol/ recreational drugs; **H**ome environment and support; **O**ccupation and impact on life		2
Closes consultation appropriately allowing the patient to ask any questions		1
Presentation: structured, concise		2
Appropriate Differential Diagnosis ± Investigations ± Management Plan		3
Examiner mark – professionalism and rapport		5
Patient mark – professionalism and rapport		5

Consultation	Presentation	Global marks patient	Global marks examiner	Total
30	5	5	5	45

55F with stress incontinence

HPC	Menopausal patient with 6 months history of incontinence. Associated with stress such as sneezing or laughter. Very distressing for patient. Reports significant negative impact on quality of life, finds herself hesitant to go to work. Wears pads and adult diapers to prevent staining. Complaining of rash in genital area, which she says is very sore and itchy. Says her genital area smells bad, despite her daily use of antibiotic soap. Exercises regularly but less recently as concerned she is going to wee herself. No dysuria, no infective symptoms. No foreign travels. STI screen negative.
PMHx	2 C-sections, 1 vaginal delivery, fit and healthy.
DHx	NKDA, Nil regular
FHx	Nil acute
SHx	Lives with husband and kids. Works as sales assistant in clothing store, on her feet all day. No smoking history, little alcohol (usually on weekend)
ICE	"I can't continue like this anymore, doctor. This is slowing me down too much. I'm not old enough for diapers. They make me feel senile. What can you do to help me?"
Ix	FBC, U&E, CRP, Bladder can, USS KUB, Stress test, consider cystoscopy if concerned
Dx	Urethral atrophy secondary to menopause
Tx	Pelvic floor exercises, HRT to prevent further atrophy

35F with incontinence

HPC	8 months history of increased frequency and incontinence. Not been a problem before. Delivered 2nd child 8 months ago. Two vaginal deliveries. Some trauma during delivery, but no significant blood loss or injury. No prolapse. Finds she needs to go more often, usually 8 times per day or more, especially during the night. Incontinence at different times during the day. No obvious trigger, describes small leakage following micturition. No infective symptoms, negative urine dip, no polydipsia, no weight gain. No SOB, chest pain or abdominal pain. No flank pains. No constipation or diarrhoea.
PMHx	Post-natal depression after 1st child, not after second. Gestational diabetes during both.
DHx	NKDA, nil regular.
FHx	Mother had stroke age 70
SHx	Housewife, mother of 2. No smoking. Lives with husband. Occasional alcohol intake
ICE	"Doctor, do you think this is because of my children? My mother in law had the same thing."
Ix	Bimanual examination, bladder scan.
Dx	Urged incontinence due to post-delivery pelvic floor weakness
Tx	Pelvic floor exercises, anticholinergics for difficult cases

75M with 4 days of incontinence

HPC	Patient with 4 days of urinary incontinence. Had elective hip replacement 2 weeks ago. Was fine before. No complications during surgery, good recovery. Painful. Has noticed that his abdomen is very distended and feels sore to touch. Says his stomach has been more grumbly than usual. Has not opened his bowel for 10 days. Some small amounts of diarrhoea. Surgical wounds healing well without any discharge from the wound, mobilizing independently. patient reports decreased appetite and thirst. Passing wind. He has also noticed some breathing difficulty but denies CP or fever. No dysuria.
PMHx	HTN, Arthritis
DHx	Codeine, Tramadol (since surgery), bisoprolol, ramipril. NKDA
FHx	Adopted. Parents unknown.
SHx	Retired police officer. Lives alone at home. Independent. Non-smoker. Alcohol 2 pints per day.
ICE	"I'm concerned that something went wrong during the surgery and the surgeons are not telling me. Do you think they could have cut a nerve? Is it going to be like this forever?"
Ix	FBC, U&E, CRP, LFT, PR, urine MSU and C/S, Bladder flow cytometry, Bladder scan
Dx	Urinary retention with overflow incontinence secondary to opiate induced constipation
Tx	Catheter to drain bladder, relieve constipation with enema, suppository followed by laxatives, alternative form of analgesia

URINARY RETENTION
GENERAL FRAMEWORK

<u>**"WIPE"**</u> – Introduce yourself, whilst gaining consent
- Wash hands
- Introduce self – "Hello, my name is X and I am a medical student"
- Patient details – "Could I ask your full name and age?"
- Explain – I have been asked to speak with you about what brings you in, would that be alright?

<u>**Open**</u>
- I understand you've have some trouble passing urine, do you mind telling me about what's been going on?
- Clarify

<u>**Timeline**</u>
1. When did this difficulty urinating start? Did anything happen around then?
2. Was it something that started suddenly or that you gradually noticed?
3. Does it come and go or is it a daily problem?
4. Has it been getting harder and harder to pass urine?
5. Have you ever had a problem like this before?

<u>**Symptoms**</u>
- **Retention**
  - ➢ How often do you manage to go? More or less that you used to?
  - ➢ How often do you feel like you want to go?
- **Urine**
  - ➢ Have you noticed any change in the smell of the urine?
  - ➢ What about the colour of the urine?
  - ➢ Have you seen any blood in your urine? How much? How often?
  - ➢ Have you noticed any foaminess or sediment?
- **Lower Urinary Tract Symptoms**
  - ➢ Do you struggle to initiate the stream of urine? Once you begin urinating, is it a continuous flow? Do you experience any dribbling of urine at the end? Do you ever find that you want to go again after you've just been?

<u>**Systems**</u>
- **Neurological** – Have you had a headache? Noticed a change in any of your senses? And what about any weakness or altered sensation?
- **Genitourinary** –How have the waterworks been? Have you had any pain on passing urine? Have you been passing urine more/ less often?
- **Anxiety** – Would you consider yourself an anxious person? Do you think this could be related to anxiety at all?
- **Constitutional** – How has your appetite been? Have you noticed a change in weight? Have you been feeling tired recently? Have you had a fever? Night-sweats?

<u>**ICE**</u>
- You've given me a lot of information, thank you. I'd like to hear a little about what you think could be going on. Do you have any idea?
- Is there anything that's particularly concerning you that you'd like to discuss?
- What exactly are you looking for today, resolution or reassurance?

PMHx
- Do you have any medical conditions?
- Ask a few specific questions to show that you're thinking about different causes
- Specifically, I'd like to ask if you've ever been diagnosed with:
  - Kidney problems? Prostate problems? Cancer? Neurological problems? Parkinson's Disease ?

DHx
- On any medication? Any doses of medication changed?
  - Specifically ask: Antidepressants (TCAs)? Asthma/ COPD inhalers? Antihistamines? (Anticholinergic properties = urinary retention)
- Any allergies?

FHx
- Any conditions run in the family? Specifically, I'd like to ask about kidney or prostate problems? Cancer? Neurological conditions?
- Has anyone in the family ever had problems with urination similar to the ones you're experiencing now?

SHx –
- Smoking/ Alcohol/ Recreational drugs
- Home environment? Support?
- Occupation – impact on life and on occupation?

Summarise and Thank
- I'd just like to summarise back to you to make sure I haven't missed anything
- Is there anything you'd like to talk about that we haven't quite addressed?
- Thank you for talking to me and I wish you all the best

Top Tip! Remember that acute retention is extremely painful, but chronic retention is painless.

Differential Diagnosis

	Diagnosis	Features In History	Features In Investigations	Management
STRUCTURAL OBSTRUCTION	BPH	Elderly men. Nocturia, frequency, small volume, difficulty initiating, poor stream, terminal dribbling, straining to pass. Gradual onset, no red flags.	Exam: Bladder may be palpable. DRE: enlarged smooth symmetrical prostate. Bloods: PSA for cancer.	Conservative: watch and wait. Medical: Tamsulosin, finasteride. Surgical: TURP
	Prostate Cancer	LUTS symptoms as in BPH with associated red flags (weight loss, anorexia, lethargy, erectile dysfunction, back pain indicates mets)	Exam: enlarged, hard, nodular prostate. Bloods: raised PSA, raised ALP in mets. Gleason score >7 is high risk.	Watchful waiting Radical surgery Adjunctive and palliative treatment of symptoms.
	Urethral Stricture	Difficulty initiating, intermittent stream, incomplete voiding, terminal dribbling. History of STI (gonococcal), recent catheter/long term, urethritis, BPH.	Normal examination – perhaps enlarged prostate on DRE. USS / cystourethroscopy / urethrogram shows stricture.	No medical therapy. Urethral dilatation or internal urethrotomy or urethral stent depending on cause and severity.
NEUROGENIC	Drugs	Retention of urine following new medication / increase in dose of anti-cholinergics (TCAs, anti-psychotics, anti-histamines, anti-muscarinic inhalers, atropine)	Exam: palpable bladder, may be tender. No findings on urine dip or bloods.	Withdraw / replace / reduce causative medication.
	Stroke / MS / PD	Urgency to go is main problem, cannot hold urine. Complicated by cognitive impairment in elderly.	Signs of underlying cause. Urine dip: NAD	Underlying cause.

Also consider: Psychogenic Retention

Investigations

Examination	Abdominal examination, DRE for prostate.
Bedside	Urine dip
Bloods	FBC, U&E, PSA, ALP, bone profile
Imaging	Bladder scan, urethrogram
Special	Cystoscopy

Marking Criteria Retention	Marks	
	Awarded	**Available**
Washes hands at the start of the station		1
Introduces themselves – Including First name, last name and role		1
Patient details confirmed: Full name, Age/ D.O.B.		1
Explains purpose of consultation		1
Open question about what brings the patient in today + Clarification of any ambiguity		1
Timeline allows a clear understanding of onset and progression - Onset/ Circumstance - Sudden vs. gradual - Fluctuations - Progression - Past episodes		3

Symptoms elicited are relevant and clearly directed at either arriving at a diagnosis or excluding other plausible diagnoses
- Retention
   o How often do you go? How often do you feel like going?
- Urine
   o Smell; Appearance; Blood; Foaminess/ sediment
- LUTS
		5

Systems queried are relevant to the complaint and adequate questions are asked for each symptom - Neurological; Genitourinary; Anxiety; Constitutional		5
Explores **Ideas, Concerns and Expectations**		3
Elicits relevant **Past Medical History** - Kidney problems; Prostate problems; Cancer; Neurological problems; PD		2
Elicits relevant **Drug History** including **Allergies**		2
Elicits relevant **Family History**		2
Elicits relevant **Social History** – including Smoking/ alcohol/ recreational drugs; **H**ome environment and support; **O**ccupation and impact on life		2
Closes consultation appropriately allowing the patient to ask any questions		1
Presentation: structured, concise		2
Appropriate Differential Diagnosis ± Investigations ± Management Plan		3
Examiner mark – professionalism and rapport		5
Patient mark – professionalism and rapport		5

Consultation	Presentation	Global marks patient	Global marks examiner	Total
$\overline{30}$	$\overline{5}$	$\overline{5}$	$\overline{5}$	$\overline{45}$

30M with urinary retention

HPC	Patient with 3 months history of worsening hesitancy and incomplete voiding. Reports mild abdominal pain, especially in the peri-umbilical area. Increased nocturnal frequency. Also describing mild incontinence of urine. Reports penile discharge and itching over last 6 months. Also reports burning sensation when passing water. No dysuria or haematuria. No flank pain, no infective symptom. No diarrhoea, no constipation. No fever, join pain/swelling or rash. It is not of major concern for him to go and see doctor. Reports foreign travel over the past 12 months, mainly to Asia, including Thailand, where he had unprotected sex with multiple prostitutes.
PMHx	Genital herpes
DHx	NKDA, nil regular. Sildenafil on occasion.
FHx	Nil relevant
SHx	Works for technology manufacturer. Married, two kids. Drinks socially, smokes on occasion. Used cocaine in the past on business trips.
ICE	"Doctor, I need to figure out what's going on. I'm constantly worried that I'm going to pee in my pants, and the dribbling makes me smell of urine which keeps me from interacting with clients."
Ix	FBC, U&E, LFT, bladder scan, PR, culture/microscopy of discharge, STI screen, HIV tests
Dx	Chronic urinary retention secondary to gonorrhoeal rosary-bead strictures.
Tx	Catheterization to relieve retention, ceftriaxone and dilatation of strictures as definitive treatment

75M with urinary retention

HPC	Presents with long term history of worsening hesitancy, nocturia and increasing frequency. Finds it difficult to urinate standing due to poor pressure. Unable to fully void. Feels as if the penis is blocked. Sometimes painful on initiation of micturition. Also reports some involuntary urination. Has pain in lower abdomen and feels sore. Reports no flank pain, no fevers or confusion. Had noticed dysuria on rare occasions only. No diarrhoea, constipation, nausea, vomiting, night sweats or weight loss. Reports recurring UTIs over the last 2 years, never had any problems in the past.
PMHx	Triple CABG 2 years ago, HTN
DHx	Aspirin, Bisoprolol, Ramipril, Simvastatin. NKDA
SHx	Retired car mechanic, lives with wife in the house. Independent. 3 children.
FHx	Mother diagnosed with bowel cancer age 75, died age 77
ICE	"Doctor, I'm concerned that I have cancer. My mom was diagnosed when she was my age and was dead 2 years after. I want to spend some time with my grandkids."
Ix	PS, FBC, U&E, LFT, CRP, Urine dip, PR, MRI
Dx	Benign prostatic hyperplasia
Tx	5-alpha-reducetase inhibitors, TURP, catheterization if retention.

55F with urinary retention.

HPC	Patient with gradual onset increased frequency of micturition and incontinence. Small amounts only. Independent of time, both during day and night. Reports abdominal pain, constipation, dysuria. Noted weight gain, but ascribed this to age. Feels her abdomen is bit bloated/distended and feels sore in lower abdomen. Says she tends to avoid wearing trousers as the waist band is uncomfortable. She has had frequent UTIs and bladder infections in the past. Usually treated with antibiotics. No infective symptoms, no fever, tachycardia or tachypnoea. No coughs or colds. No chest pain, no SOB.
PMHx	MS
DHx	NKDA, nil regular, previous courses of steroids for acute MS attacks
FHx	Nil relevant.
SHx	Part-time teacher, used to be full time, but cut down due to MS, Mother of 2, married. Non-smoker, no alcohol. Mobile and independent for daily activities.
ICE	"Doctor, I'm concerned that this is my MS getting worse. Am I going to need to have a catheter all the time or am I going to remain fully incontinent? How is that going to affect my work?"
Ix	FBC, U&E, CRP, detrusor muscle electromyogram
Dx	Bladder sphincter dyssynergia
Tx	Catheterize to drain, surgery or Botulinum A injections if not for surgery. Long term catheter.

HAEMATURIA
GENERAL FRAMEWORK

"WIPE" – Introduce yourself, whilst gaining consent
- Wash hands
- Introduce self – "Hello, my name is X and I am a medical student"
- Patient details – "Could I ask your full name and age?"
- Explain – "I have been asked to speak with you about what brings you in, would that be alright?"

Open
- I understand you've passed some blood in your urine, which I can imagine must have been quite distressing for you. Do you mind telling me about that?
- **Clarify** – Can I clarify whether the blood is definitely coming with the urine or could it be due to menstruation or coming from the back passage, for example?

Timeline
1. When did you first notice this? Did anything happen around then? E.g. Trauma
2. Was it something you suddenly noticed or gradually became aware of?
3. Does it come and go or do you see blood every time you pass urine?
4. Have you been passing increasing amounts of urine?
5. Have you ever had anything like this before?

Symptoms
- **Urine**
  - ➤ **Colour** – What colour is the urine? Red/ Orange?
  - ➤ **Amount** – How much blood roughly if you had to estimate? Splatter? Spoonful? Cupful?
  - ➤ **Distribution** – Do you notice blood at the start (urethra), throughout (kidneys, ureters, bladder), or end (prostate) of the stream of urine?
  - ➤ **Smell** – is there a particularly foul smell to the urine?
  - ➤ **Foaminess/ Sediment** – Have you noticed any foaminess or sediment?
- **Discharge** – Have you noticed any discharge from your penis/ vagina?
- **Rashes** – Have you noticed any rashes or blisters in your penis/ vagina?
- **Illness** – Have you been ill recently?
- **Pain** – Any pain in the tummy area?
- **Lower Urinary Tract Symptoms**
  - ➤ Do you struggle to initiate the stream of urine? Once you begin urinating, is it a continuous flow? Do you experience any dribbling of urine at the end? Do you ever find that you want to go again after you've just been?
- **Associated**
- **Renal failure** – any weight gain? Swollen ankles?
- **Glomerulonephritis** – recently had a sore throat? Any rashes or sore joints?
- **Pulmonary-renal conditions** – recently coughed up any blood?
- **Trauma** – any trauma to your stomach or groin?
- **Travel** – any foreign travel (Esp. Africa – Schistosomiasis in Lake Malawi)

Systems
- **Genitourinary** –How have the waterworks been? Have you had any pain on passing urine? Have you been passing urine more/ less often? Do you ever leak urine? Feel an urgent need to pass urine?
- **Musculoskeletal** – Have you had any back or joint pain? Any stiffness?
- **Gynaecological** – Are you sexually active? Is there any chance you could be pregnant? When was your last menstrual period?
- **Constitutional** – How has your appetite been? Have you noticed a change in weight? Have you been feeling tired recently? Have you had a fever? Night-sweats?

ICE
- You've given me a lot of information, thank you. I'd like to hear a little about what you think could be going on. Do you have any idea?
- Is there anything that's particularly concerning you that you'd like to discuss?
- What exactly are you looking for today, resolution or reassurance?

PMHx
- Do you have any medical conditions?
- Ask a few specific questions to show that you're thinking about different causes
- Specifically, I'd like to ask if you've ever been diagnosed with:
  - ➢ A urinary tract infection? A sexually transmitted infection? Bladder problems? Prostate problems? Kidney problems/ stones? Cancer? Tuberculosis?

DHx
- On any medication? Any doses of medication changed?
  - ➢ Specifically ask: Tuberculosis medication? This may seem like an unrelated question but do you drink beetroot juice?
- Any allergies?

FHx
- Any conditions run in the family? Specifically, I'd like to ask about Kidney or bladder problems? Bleeding problems?
- Has anyone in the family ever had symptoms similar to the ones you're experiencing?

SHx
- Smoking/ Alcohol/ Recreational drugs (Especially KETAMINE)
- Home environment? Support?
- Occupation (Especially RUBBER/ DYE) – impact on life and on occupation?

Summarise and Thank
- I'd just like to summarise back to you to make sure I haven't missed anything
- Is there anything you'd like to talk about that we haven't quite addressed?
- Thank you for talking to me and I wish you all the best

Investigations

Examination	Abdominal examination, DRE, genital examination
Bedside	Temperature, urine dip, BM
Bloods	FBC, U&E, CRP, CK, LDH,
Imaging	USS KUB
Special	Swabs, urine MC&S, cystoscopy

Top Tip! Microscopic haematuria and frank haematuria have different causes – make sure you take the time to understand if the blood is visible easily (frank) or noticed it when testing their urine (e.g. at GP surgery etc)

Differential Diagnosis

	Diagnosis	Features In History	Features In Investigations	Management
INTRINSIC TO URINARY TRACT	**Trauma**	Bloody urine following trauma to the urinary tract e.g. catheter, RTA, fall, violence. Sudden onset after, associated with pain. Ensure there are no red flags present.	Full primary and secondary survey in RTA / violence / fall to look for injury. Urine dip: blood – may be visible Bleed on USS KUB	Most commonly catheter – remove and trial of void.
	Cancer (bladder / prostate)	Frank haematuria, persisting after UTI treatment. Weight loss, anorexia, Risk factors are: male, >45, FH, smoking	Urine dip: blood, perhaps leucocytes. Cystoscopy: cancer confirm on biopsy. CT abdomen-pelvis to stage.	2 week wait referral to urology for investigation of cancer.
	UTI	Dysuria, frequency, small amounts of urine. Associated with fevers, myalgia, feeling unwell.	Foul smelling urine. Urine dip: positive leucocytes and nitrites. Bloods: raised WCC and CRP. Organisms on gram stain and culture.	Antibiotics e.g. trimethoprim or nitrofurantoin. Also assess features of sepsis and need for fluid resuscitation.
	Renal Colic	Sudden severe pain from "loin to groin" on one side, find it hard to get comfortable, haematuria, previous history of kidney stones. Fever and rigors may indicate pyelonephritis.	Tender over renal angle. Blood leucocytes on urine dip. USS KUB shows stone in ureter	Stones < 5mm likely pass spontaneously. >5mm likely to need urological intervention. Tamsulosin can help.
EXTRINSIC TO URINARY TRACT	**Rhabdomyolysis**	Triad: myalgia, generalised weakness and darkened urine. Normally after prolonged immobilisation, long lie after a fall or excessive exertion	Bloods: Raised CK (peak 24-36h). May show AKI, hyperkalaemia, raised LDH,	Rehydration is mainstay and measure urine output, monitor for DIC.
	Exercise Induced	Red urine after intense physical activity (e.g. running marathon) or contact sports. No other signs of systemic upset or infection, no red flags.	Blood on urine dip with no findings on examination or imaging.	Nil, reassure.
	STI	Haematuria associated with urethral discharge. History of risky sexual activity (multiple partners, no barrier contraception, previous STIs).	Exam: urethral discharge. Swabs positive for gonorrhoea / chlamydia most commonly.	Antibiotic treatment 1g azithromycin stat (and ceftriaxone if gonococcal), patient education and contact tracing.

Also consider:
- Beeturia (single red episode after a lot of beetroot).
- Gynaecological conditions e.g. placenta Praevia, menstruation
- Drugs e.g. Rifampicin.
- Parasitic infections e.g. schistosomiasis (if positive travel history)

Marking Criteria Haematuria	Marks	
	Awarded	Available
Washes hands at the start of the station		1
Introduces themselves – Including First name, last name and role		1
Patient details confirmed: Full name, Age/ D.O.B.		1
Explains purpose of consultation		1
Open question about what brings the patient in today + Clarification of any ambiguity – Ex. blood definitely coming with urine vs. from menstruation/ back passage?		1
Timeline allows a clear understanding of onset and progression - Onset/ Circumstance - Sudden vs. gradual - Fluctuations - Progression - Past episodes		3

Symptoms elicited are relevant and clearly directed at either arriving at a diagnosis or excluding other plausible diagnoses
- Urine
   o Colour; Amount; Distribution blood; Smell; Foaminess/ sediment
- Discharge
- Rashes
- Illness
- LUTS
- Associated
   o Renal failure; GN; Pulmonary-Renal conditions; Trauma; Travel
		5

Systems queried are relevant to the complaint and adequate questions are asked for each symptom - Genitourinary; Musculoskeletal; Gynaecological; Constitutional		5
Explores **Ideas, Concerns and Expectations**		3
Elicits relevant **Past Medical History** - UTI; STI; Bladder problems; Prostate problems; Kidney problems/ stones; Cancer; TB		2
Elicits relevant **Drug History** including **Allergies**		2
Elicits relevant **Family History**		2
Elicits relevant **Social History** – including Smoking/ alcohol/ recreational drugs; **H**ome environment and support; **O**ccupation and impact on life		2
Closes consultation appropriately allowing the patient to ask any questions		1
Presentation: structured, concise		2
Appropriate Differential Diagnosis ± Investigations ± Management Plan		3
Examiner mark – professionalism and rapport		5
Patient mark – professionalism and rapport		5

Consultation	Presentation	Global marks patient	Global marks examiner	Total
$\overline{30}$	$\overline{5}$	$\overline{5}$	$\overline{5}$	$\overline{45}$

35M with 3 week history of red urine

HPC	Patient presents with 3-week History of red urine. Sudden onset. Patient does not report any trauma. No dysuria. He does report a chronic cough and some weight loss. Had some haemoptysis in the past, but not for some time. Cough is improving. Currently no infective symptoms, however he remembers having severe night sweats and nocturnal fevers 3 weeks ago. No dizziness, not palpitations, no SOB, no CP. Some vomiting, nausea and diarrhoea over the past weeks. Travelled regularly to Asia in the past for business. Patient does not remember the exact diagnosis, but says he was told it was a pretty serious illness. Reports having been asked if he had been vaccinated as a child at school and if he had a scar on his arm.
PMHx	Recently diagnosed pulmonary tuberculosis
DHx	Rifampicin, Isoniazid, Ethambutol, pyrazinamide and pyridoxine. NKDA
SHx	Works for NGO, drinks 4 units of alcohol per day. No IVDU, smoked cannabis in the past.
FHx	Nil
ICE	"Doctor, I'm just worried that something is wrong with my kidneys."
Ix	FBC, U&E, LFT, CRP, Sputum culture, Urine dip, consider USS KUB
Dx	Rifampicin side-effect.
Tx	Reassurance. No treatment needed, Rifampicin side-effect is harmless and non-toxic.

60M with 3 months of haematuria

HPC	Patient complaining of 3 months history of haematuria. Denies any infective symptoms. No fevers, loin pain, weight loss or night sweats. Some problems passing urine, but ongoing issue for a long time. Previous doctors said "Normal for a man your age". Problems passing urine, feels like he passes a little and then has to go again, complaining of "dribble". No impotence. No dysuria, no flank pain. No fever, abdominal pain, diarrhoea or vomiting. No cough or constipation. No PR bleed. Feels some pain behind right testicle, especially when he needs to pass water. Relieved when passing water. Pain is worst in the morning before he empties his bladder and his bowels.
PMHx	HTN, T2DM - diet controlled.
DHx	Bisoprolol, Aspirin, NKDA
FHx	Cardiac history on father's side. Dad had MI age 70
SHx	Teacher. Drinks 8 units per day. Lifelong non-smoker.
ICE	"Doctor, I'm concerned that this has something to do with my testes. Could it be cancer?"
Ix	FBC, U&E, LFT, PR exam, USS prostate, consider MRI, biopsy, PSA
Dx	Prostate Cancer
Tx	Radiotherapy or surgery, consider 5-alpha-reductase-inhibitors

40F with dysuria and haematuria

HPC	4-day history of gradually worsening dysuria. 1-day history of haematuria. Patient complaining of flank pain, fevers and tachycardia. She feels cold, dizzy and think his heart is racing more than usual. She feels very unwell and struggling to focus. Denies any confusion but feels very distressed and anxious. She is noticing abdominal pain, more on the back. Pain started gradually as a burning sensation when passing water, now much worse and includes flanks. Worse on right side, radiating to the back. Patient feels nauseous and says she feels like she is going to be sick. No vomiting, no diarrhoea, no constipation.
PMHx	Recurrent UTIs, C-section when delivering 2nd child 10 years ago.
DHx	NKDA, Mirena coil.
FHx	Father diagnosed with bladder cancer in 60s
SHx	Works as sales rep. Travels a lot. Non-smoker. Drinks 2 glasses of red wine on weekend.
ICE	"This feels nothing like the UTIs I normally get. I don't know what's going on, I feel very unwell."
Ix	FBC, CRP, U&E, LFT, Urine dip, USS KUB, consider CT renal tract if stable, blood and urine culture for sensitivity,
Dx	Pyelonephritis
Tx	Follow local antibiotic guidelines, usually, amoxicillin IV, gentamicin IV, fluid resuscitation as appropriate, paracetamol, consider diclofenac for renal colic type pain.

NOCTURIA & POLYURIA
GENERAL FRAMEWORK

"WIPE" – Introduce yourself, whilst gaining consent
- Wash hands
- Introduce self – "Hello, my name is X and I am a medical student"
- Patient details – "Could I ask your full name and age?"
- Explain – "I have been asked to speak with you about what brings you in, would that be alright?"

Open
- I understand you've been passing more urine than usual/ at night than usual, do you mind telling me about what's been going on?
- Clarify – Can I just clarify whether you've been passing a greater amount of urine or simply that you're passing urine more often but smaller amounts?

Timeline
1. When did you first notice this change in your waterworks? Did anything happen around then?
2. Was it something that happened suddenly or something you gradually grew aware of?
3. Does this come and go or do you pass large amounts of urine all the time?
4. Have you been passing increasing amounts of urine?
5. Have you ever had a problem like this before?

Symptoms
- **Urine**
  - ➤ Have you noticed any change the smell of the urine?
  - ➤ Colour of the urine? (Pale = dilute in DM, DI)
  - ➤ Have you seen any blood in the urine? How much? How often?
  - ➤ Have you noticed any foaminess or sediment?
- **Discharge** – Have you noticed any discharge from your penis/ vagina?
- **Rashes** – Have you noticed any rashes or blisters in your penis/ vagina?
- **Illness** – Have you been ill recently?
- **Lower Urinary Tract Symptoms**
  - ➤ Do you struggle to initiate the stream of urine? Once you begin urinating, is it a continuous flow? Do you experience any dribbling of urine at the end? Do you ever find that you want to go again after you've just been?

Systems
- **Cardiovascular** – Did you have any chest pain? Palpitations? SOB? Do you feel breathless lying down or at night? Do you often get ankle/ lower back swelling?
- **Genitourinary** –How have the waterworks been? Have you had any pain on passing urine? Have you noticed any changes in the colour of the urine? Have you been passing urine more/ less often? Do you ever leak urine? Feel an urgent need to pass urine?
- **Anxiety** – Would you consider yourself to be an anxious person? Do you think it could be related?
- **Constitutional** – How has your appetite been? Have you noticed a change in weight? Have you been feeling tired recently? Have you had a fever? Night-sweats?

ICE
- You've given me a lot of information, thank you. I'd like to hear a little about what you think could be going on. Do you have any idea?
- Is there anything that's particularly concerning you that you'd like to discuss?
- What exactly are you looking for today, resolution or reassurance?

PMHx
- Do you have any medical conditions?
- Ask a few specific questions to show that you're thinking about different causes
- Specifically, I'd like to ask if you've ever been diagnosed with:
  - Something called Diabetes mellitus? Diabetes insipidus? Urinary tract infections? Prostate problems? Kidney problems? Kidney stones? Sexually transmitted infections? Any recent procedures (cystoscopy, renal surgery, etc.)?

DHx
- On any medication? Any doses of medication changed?
  - Specifically ask: Diuretics (ACE-i)? Long-term antibiotics?
- Any allergies?

FHx
- Any conditions run in the family? Specifically, I'd like to ask about Kidney or bladder problems? Diabetes mellitus? Diabetes insipidus?
- Has anyone in the family ever had symptoms similar to the ones you're experiencing?

SHx –
- Smoking/ Alcohol/ Recreational drugs
- Home environment? Support?
- Occupation – impact on life and on occupation?

Summarise and Thank
- I'd just like to summarise back to you to make sure I haven't missed anything
- Is there anything you'd like to talk about that we haven't quite addressed?
- Thank you for talking to me and I wish you all the best

Investigations

Examination	Abdominal exam, genital examination if indicated
Bedside	Urine dip, BP, blood glucose
Bloods	U&E, FBC, HbA1c, serum osmolality
Imaging	USS KUB
Special	Urine sodium, protein:creatinine ratio and osmolality. 24hour urinary sodium, water deprivation test

Differential Diagnosis

	Diagnosis	Features In History	Features In Investigations	Management
INCREASED WATER INTAKE	**Diabetes Mellitus**	Polyuria, polydipsia, tiredness, weight loss, FH of DM, personal history of other autoimmune diseases.	Exam: may seem tired, dehydrated. Urine dip: glucose. Bloods: high glucose, HbA1c.	Rehydration, check for DKA and treat if present as emergency. T1DM: insulin T2DM: oral hypoglycaemics. Endocrinology referral.
	Diabetes Insipidus	Polyuria (3-20L), polydipsia, nocturia. May have history of pituitary/ hypothalamic surgery or trauma.	Don't tend to be dehydrated Reduced urine osmolality, preserved/raised plasma osmolality. Vasopressin test for neurogenic vs nephrogenic (will treat neurogenic).	Fluid replacement if needed. Neurogenic DI: desmopressin. Nephrogenic DI: treat underlying cause if known. NSAIDS, diuretics are alternatives.
	Psychogenic Polydipsia	Excessive urination and excessive fluid intake. No dysuria, weight loss. Generally no systemic symptoms unless hyponatraemic. More common in schizophrenia.	Examination: no findings. Fluid deprivation test: concentrated urine produced.	Dietary control and psychological support.
NORMAL WATER INTAKE	**UTI**	Dysuria, frequency, small amounts of urine. Associated with fevers, myalgia, feeling unwell.	Foul smelling urine. Urine dip: positive leucocytes and nitrites. Bloods: raised WCC and CRP	Antibiotics – trimethoprim or nitrofurantoin. Also assess features of sepsis and need for fluid resuscitation.
	Diuretics	Polyuria of new onset after the start of a new "blood pressure tablet". Worse in the hours after tablet, no systemic symptoms. May also have incontinence or nocturia with this.	No specific findings on examination. May be hypertensive. No abdominal findings. Bloods: look out for hypokalaemia in loop and thiazide diuretics.	Reassure and reduce dose if not coping. Treat any complications of diuretic use.

Also Consider: Fanconi's Syndrome

Marking Criteria Nocturia/ Polyuria	Marks	
	Awarded	Available
Washes hands at the start of the station		1
Introduces themselves – Including First name, last name and role		1
Patient details confirmed: Full name, Age/ D.O.B.		1
Explains purpose of consultation		1
Open question about what brings the patient in today + Clarification of any ambiguity – Ex. greater amount of urine vs small amounts more often		1
Timeline allows a clear understanding of onset and progression - Onset/ Circumstance - Sudden vs. gradual - Fluctuations - Progression - Past episodes		3
Symptoms elicited are relevant and clearly directed at either arriving at a diagnosis or excluding other plausible diagnoses - Urine o Colour; Amount; Smell; Blood; Foaminess/ sediment - Discharge - Rashes - Illness - LUTS		5
Systems queried are relevant to the complaint and adequate questions are asked for each symptom - Cardiovascular; Genitourinary; Anxiety; Constitutional		5
Explores **Ideas, Concerns and Expectations**		3
Elicits relevant **Past Medical History** - DM; DI; UTI; STI; Prostate problems; Kidney problems; Recent procedures (Ex. cystoscopy, renal surgery, etc.)		2
Elicits relevant **Drug History** including **Allergies**		2
Elicits relevant **Family History**		2
Elicits relevant **Social History** – including Smoking/ alcohol/ recreational drugs; **H**ome environment and support; **O**ccupation and impact on life		2
Closes consultation appropriately allowing the patient to ask any questions		1
Presentation: structured, concise		2
Appropriate Differential Diagnosis ± Investigations ± Management Plan		3
Examiner mark – professionalism and rapport		5
Patient mark – professionalism and rapport		5

Consultation	Presentation	Global marks patient	Global marks examiner	Total
30	5	5	5	45

25F with Polyuria

HPC	Patient with 1-month history of polyuria. Delivered he first child not 1 months ago, was troubled with high urine output during pregnancy, but ascribed that to the baby pressing the bladder. Drinks 5-7 l of iced water a day, as well as some coffee, juice and soft drinks, finds herself thirsty all the time. Says she sleeps well, considering her 4-week-old baby and despite waking up a few times during the night to pass urine. Reports no abdominal pain, no headache, no haematuria, no dysuria, no infective symptoms. No post-partum complications. Normal delivery. Baby is fit and well. No palpitations, no chest pain, no foreign travel.
PMHx	Broken arm age 7
FHx	Nil relevant
DHx	NKDA, was on depot injections prior to pregnancy.
SHx	Lives with husband and baby. Used to work in retail. No alcohol, no smoking.
ICE	"I am so incredibly busy taking care of the baby, I can't be running to the toilet all the time."
Ix	U&E,TFT, cortisol, serum & urine osmolality, blood sugar, fluid deprivation test, MRI pituitary
Dx	Diabetes Insipidus
Tx	Desmopressin, careful monitoring of urine production and osmolality. Monitor serum sodium.

50M with Nocturia

HPC	Patient with nocturia over last few months. Finds himself getting up almost every hour and then has difficulties falling back asleep. He also finds that he is thirstier than he used to be. He thinks his urine has a sweet smell to it. Patient is obese and has been struggling with his weight for some time but has lost 2 kg in last few weeks. Finds it difficult to exercise as he lacks energy and quickly get short of breath. Also feels like others are judging him for his body. Ashamed to leave the house. Tends to avoid public transport. Reports no dysuria now but has noticed increased tendency to have thrush, no haematuria, and no voiding problems. No fever, cough, chest pain, swollen ankles, palpitations, abdomen pain or bowel change.
PMHx	Obesity
DHx	Nil regular, NKDA
FHx	Father had heart attack age 68
SHx	Works as delivery driver. Drinks occasionally, smokes for 20 years.
ICE	"Doctor, it's becoming harder and harder to cope with this. I'm not sleeping enough; I almost crashed my delivery truck the other day because I fell asleep behind the wheel."
Ix	FBC, U&E, LFT, HbA1c, blood sugar levels, urine dip
Dx	Type 2 Diabetes Mellitus
Tx	Diet and life style advice, weight management, blood sugar lowering medications (oral to start with). Will need education, retinal screening, feet care advice. DVLA advice

40 years old male with polyuria

HPC	Patient with gradual onset of polyuria over several months. Also complaining of bone pain and and muscle weakness. He has sustained 3 fractures falling over at home in the last nine months. He says his urine always looks very foamy and has a sweet honey like smell. He also says that he feels thirstier than usually.
PMHx	HIV and depression
DHx	NKDA, on tenofovir and didanosine, prozac and recent course of doxycycline.
FHx	Father had 3 heart attacks, first age 45
SHx	Lives with partner, works in bank. Non-smoker, social alcohol consumption
ICE	"I feel like I'm peeing all the time & I hurt all over. I don't know what to do anymore, doctor. "
Dx	Fanconi syndrome
Ix	FBC, U&E, LFT, urine dip, urine analysis for solutes, USS KUB, ABG for pH
Tx	Bone protection with Vitamin D and calcium and phosphate supplementation. Balance serum acidity with bicarbonate, consider potassium supplementation if K low.

GENERAL HISTORIES

These general histories have a broad range of DDx which often makes it hard to ask all relevant questions in the time-pressured setting of an OSCE. For each of the following presenting complaints, I have included a list of common symptoms you can ask about for each condition. However, if you don't wish to memorise all of these different question sets, you can usually elicit all the relevant information and exclude most DDx by performing a brief generalised screen of the bodily SYSTEMS and being familiarised with common diagnoses.

TIREDNESS & MALAISE

"WIPE" – Introduce yourself, whilst gaining consent
- Wash hands
- Introduce self – "Hello, my name is X and I am a medical student"
- Patient details – "Could I ask your full name and age?"
- Explain – "I have been asked to speak with you about what brings you in, would that be alright?"

Open
- I understand you've been feeling tired recently. Would you mind telling me a little about what's been going on?
- **Clarification**: When you say tired, do you mean physically drained or sleepy?

Timeline
1. When did you first notice the tiredness? Did anything happen around then?
2. Did it come on suddenly or gradually?
3. Are you tired all the time or does this come and go?
4. Has the tiredness been getting worse?
5. Have you ever felt like this before?

Symptoms
- **Tiredness**
  - ➤ Is the tiredness worse at any particular **time of the day**?
  - ➤ Can you think of anything that **brings** it on? Makes it **better**?
  - ➤ How badly is this **affecting** you?
- **Remember: "ABBCCDDEE"**
  - ➤ **Anaemia** – Have you had heavy periods? Do you feel breathless?
  - ➤ **Bowels** – Have you had any bowel problems?
  - ➤ **Biological** – Have you been sleeping? Have you been eating?
  - ➤ **Cancer** – How's your appetite? Weight? Had any fevers?
  - ➤ **Chronic fatigue syndrome (Fibromyalgia)** – Had any muscle pains?
  - ➤ **Depression** – How has your mood been?
  - ➤ **Diabetes** – Have you felt particularly thirsty? Passed more urine?
  - ➤ **Endocrine (Hypothyroidism)** – Felt cold? Gained weight? Throat lump?
  - ➤ **EBV (or other infection)** – Have you been ill or had a sore throat recently?
- **General**
  - ➤ Other than tiredness, have you noticed any other changes?

ICE
- You've given me a lot of information, thank you. I'd like to hear a little about what you think could be going on. Do you have any idea?
- Is there anything that's particularly concerning you that you'd like to discuss?
- What exactly are you looking for today, resolution or reassurance?

Systems

- Consider asking about any system depending on what you have elicited so far. If you have no idea what is going on, try a quick bodily systems review:
  - ➤ **Neurological** – Have you had a headache? Noticed a change in any of your senses? And what about any weakness or altered sensation?
  - ➤ **Cardiorespiratory** – Have you had any chest pain or discomfort? Any shortness-of-breath? Any coughing?
  - ➤ **Gastrointestinal** – Have you noticed any change in your bowels?
  - ➤ **Genitourinary** – And what about the waterworks?
  - ➤ **Gynaecological** – Is there any chance you could be pregnant?
  - ➤ **Musculoskeletal** – Have you noticed any joint or pain or stiffness?
  - ➤ **Psychiatric** – How has your mood been? Have you been feeling particularly anxious?
  - ➤ **Constitutional** – Have you noticed a change in weight? Fevers? Night-sweats?

PMHx

- Do you have any medical conditions?
- Ask a few specific questions to show that you're thinking about different causes
  Specifically, I'd like to ask if you've ever been diagnosed with:
  - ➤ Something called an autoimmune disease?
  - ➤ Diabetes, thyroid problems, fibromyalgia?
  - ➤ Have you ever been diagnosed with cancer?

DHx

- Are you on any medication? Anything over-the-counter or alternative medicines?
- Have any medications been changed recently?
- Are you allergic to anything that you know of?

FHx

- Do any conditions run in the family? Consider asking specifics as for PMHx!
- Has anyone in the family ever gone through anything similar to what you're going though?

SHx

- Smoking/ Alcohol/ Recreational drugs
- Home environment? Have you been getting support to cope with everything?
- Occupation – What do you do for a living if you don't mind me asking? How has this impacted on your life and occupation?

Summarise and Thank

- I'd just like to summarise back to you to make sure I haven't missed anything
- Is there anything you'd like to talk about that we haven't quite addressed?
- Thank you for talking to me and I wish you all the best

Investigations

Examination	Full physical examination
Bedside	Urinalysis, blood glucose
Bloods	FBC, U&E, LFTs, HbA1c, TFTs, tumour markers, iron studies.
Imaging	CT CAP if cancer suspected
Special	Polysomnography, endoscopy, colonoscopy,

Differential Diagnosis

	Diagnosis	Features In History	Features In Investigations	Management
ENDOCRINE	**Diabetes Mellitus**	Polyuria, polydipsia, tiredness, weight loss, FH of DM, personal history of other autoimmune diseases.	Exam: may seem tired, dehydrated. Urine dip: glucose. Bloods: high glucose, HbA1c.	Exclude DKA. T1DM: insulin T2DM: oral hypoglycaemics. Endocrinology referral.
	Hypothyroidism	Tiredness, weight gain, cold intolerance, constipation, irregular periods, dry skin and hair. FH or personal history of autoimmune diseases.	Full examination including thyroid exam – goitre, bradycardia, slowed reflexes, dry hair. Bloods: raised TSH, low or normal T4.	Thyroxine to treat and titrate to TSH. Consider other autoimmune diseases that may also be present.
PSYCHIATRIC	**Depression**	Tiredness, lack of interest in doing things, early morning waking, low mood. Screen thoughts of deliberate self-harm and suicide. May have history of mental illness, emotional trauma. Ask about risk factors.	Nil findings on physical examination or bloods – have to screen for organic causes. Signs of depression on MSE.	Bio-psycho-social approach with advice re: diet, hydration and exercise. Psychotherapy / CBT. Medication such as SSRIs.
	Chronic Fatigue Syndrome	Fatigue for >6 months with no clear cause and associated with cognitive difficulties. Post exertional fatigue, despite sufficient sleep. May be preceded by infection trigger.	No findings on examination or blood tests. Some reports of raised viral titres (Coxsackie, HHV-6)	No proven treatments – can try exercise and supportive therapy.
OTHER	**Cancer**	B-symptoms (FLAWS): fever, lethargy, appetite loss, weight loss, sweats. May be able to pin down organ with systems review.	Full examination of all systems. Urine dip and blood tests incl. Cancer markers (CEA, PSA, CA 125, CA 19-9, AFP)	Urgent 2WW for relevant specialty, counselling and MDT approach to treatment.
	Anaemia	Gradually progressive tiredness, SOBOE, pale. Common sources – Menorrhagia PR bleeds, haematuria.	Full examination including DRE if suspected. Urine dip: haematuria. Bloods: low Hb, low iron	
	Obstructive Sleep Apnoea	Tiredness persisting for months, not rested after sleep, snoring, daytime somnolence. RF: obese, facial deformities. Ass. With HTN, IHD, DM, asthma, metabolic syndrome.	Neck circumference, raised BMI. Epworth sleepiness scale. Polysomnography (>4 respiratory events / hr)	CPAP, patient education, managing risk factors, weight loss.

Also consider:

  ➤ HIV
  ➤ Vasculitis
  ➤ Rarer Endocrine Disorders: Hypogonadism, Inborn Errors of Metabolism
  ➤ Organ Failure: Liver Cirrhosis, Heart Failure, Uraemia (secondary to renal failure)

Marking Criteria MALAISE/ TIREDNESS	Marks	
	Awarded	Available
Washed hands at the start of the station		1
Introduced themselves – Including First name, last name and role		1
Patient details confirmed: Full name, Age/ D.O.B.		1
Explained purpose of consultation		1
Open question about what brings the patient in today + Clarification of any ambiguity – E.g. Tiredness vs. malaise		1
Timeline allows a clear understanding of onset and progression - Onset/ Circumstance - Sudden vs. gradual - Fluctuations - Progression - Past episodes		3

Symptoms elicited are relevant and clearly directed at either arriving at a diagnosis or excluding other plausible diagnoses
- Tiredness variation/ triggers/ severity
- Enquires sensitively about: "**ABBCCDDEE**"
   o **A**naemia – heavy menstruation
   o **B**owel problems
   o **B**iological – poor sleep; malnutrition/ dehydration
   o **C**ancer – lack of appetite; weight loss; fevers
   o **C**hronic fatigue syndrome/ fibromyalgia – generalised muscle pains
   o **D**epression
   o **D**iabetes – polyuria and polydipsia
   o **E**ndocrine – cold intolerance/ weight gain/ goitre etc.
   o **E**BV or other infection – recent illness
- General enquiry – other than tiredness, have you noticed any other changes?
		5

Systems queried are relevant to the complaint and adequate questions are asked for each symptom - Neurological; Cardiorespiratory; Gastrointestinal; Genitourinary; Gynaecological; Musculoskeletal; Psychiatric; Constitutional		5
Explores **Ideas, Concerns and Expectations**		3
Elicits relevant **Past Medical History** - Autoimmunity; diabetes; thyroid problems; fibromyalgia; malignancy		2
Elicits relevant **Drug History** including **Allergies**		2
Elicits relevant **Family History**		2
Elicits relevant **Social History** – including Smoking/ alcohol/ recreational drugs; Home environment and support; Occupation and impact on life		2
Closes consultation appropriately allowing the patient to ask any questions		1
Presentation: structured, concise		2
Appropriate Differential Diagnosis ± Investigations ± Management Plan		3
Examiner mark – professionalism and rapport		5
Patient mark – professionalism and rapport		5

Consultation	Presentation	Global marks patient	Global marks examiner	Total
$\overline{30}$	$\overline{5}$	$\overline{5}$	$\overline{5}$	$\overline{45}$

25F presents with increasing tiredness

HPC	Patient has been feeling increasingly tired for some time. Gets particularly bad around her period, but then slowly improves after. She says she always had quiet heavy periods. This has not changed. Normally fit and well. Exercises regularly. She says she has recently changed her diet and has switched to veganism after watching a documentary about slaughterhouses. She strictly avoids all animal based food products, including food supplements. She prefers raw food. Patient denies SOB, chest pain or dizziness. Reports no nausea, vomiting, abdomen pain, weight loss or night sweats. No diarrhoea, PR or non-cycle PV bleeds. Not pregnant.
PMHx	Nil. Fit and healthy.
DHx	Hormone depot injection for contraception, occasional paracetamol for headaches.
SHx	Drinks socially, non-smoker, works as lawyer
FHx	Mother has fibroids, grandmother had hysterectomy and oophorectomy for ovarian cancer age 75
ICE	"I need to stop being so tired all the time. I can't do my job properly anymore."
Ix	FBC, peripheral blood film, Iron studies, U&E, LFT, TFT, haematinics. 2nd line investigations included OGD/Colonoscopy, bone marrow biopsy
Dx	Iron deficiency anaemia secondary to heavy periods
Tx	Iron supplement, consider Mirena coil if heavy periods are a problem

22F with 4 months history of tiredness

HPC	She has been unmotivated and generally sleepier. Finds herself sleeping more and more during the day and the staying awake during the night. She is a law student. Says her grades have been getting worse. Concerned that she will fail her degree. Feels pressured by her parents. Used to enjoy going out with her friends, hasn't done so in 6 months as she feels too stressed. She feels unmotivated to do any of the things she used to enjoy. Denies chest pain, palpitation, excessive sweating, cough, fevers, colds, foreign travel. She is not constipated and skin feels normal to her.
PMHx	Anxiety
DHx	NKDA, oral contraceptive pill, nil regular otherwise.
FHx	Grandmother diagnosed with bowel cancer age 40; grandfather has heart disease
SHx	Lives at home with her parents and siblings. Student. Single. Drinks socially. Non-smoker. No IVDU, admits having tried Ritalin 7 months ago.
ICE	"Doctor, I'm just worried that I will fail my exams. I feel so worthless and all the people around me are so smart and work so hard. I need your help so I can continue working for my degree."
Ix	FBC, U&E, TFT, Vitamin B and folate, iron studies
Dx	Depression
Tx	Cognitive behavioral therapy or anti-depressants. Be aware of increased risk of suicide when starting antidepressant. Provide safety net.

30M with 5 month history of tiredness

HPC	5 months of tiredness and generally low mood and fatigue. Patient said he feels much less energetic than he used to and has been feeling so for a while, gotten worse over the last 5 months. Reduced libido. Weight gain. Feels weaker. Gynecomastia. Increased adipose tissue deposition around thighs and belly for some time. Has problems sleeping. No fever, no coughs, no cold, no vomiting or diarrhoea. No cardiac symptoms.
PMHx	Femoral fracture 3 months ago when falling out of bed. Otherwise fit and healthy.
DHx	NKDA, zopiclone PRN.
FHx	Nil
SHx	Drinks 3 pints per day, ex-smoker. No IVDU. Works as branch manager of local bank
ICE	"I don't think I should be breaking my leg in my 30s simply by falling out of bed. Please help!"
Ix	FBC, U&E, LFT, Bone Profile, Vit D levels, TFT, coeliac screen, Free testosterone, LH and FSH level, random cortisol (and short synacthen test if necessary), CXR, pituitary MRI, DEXA scan
Dx	Hypogonadism
Tx	Lifestyle advice to improve sleep and diet, testosterone (gel, tablet/injections/depot), bone protection with bisphosphonates if DEXA positive (otherwise Vit D/Calcium), exercise.

WEIGHT LOSS
GENERAL FRAMEWORK

"WIPE" – Introduce yourself, whilst gaining consent
- Wash hands
- Introduce self – "Hello, my name is X and I am a medical student"
- Patient details – "Could I ask your full name and age?"
- Explain – "I have been asked to speak with you about what brings you in, would that be alright?"

Open
- I understand you've lost some weight recently. Do you mind telling me what's been going on?
- **± Clarification** – Can I assume this weight loss has been unintentional?

Timeline
- When did you first start losing weight? Did anything happen around then?
- Has the weight loss been sudden or gradual?
- Does your weight fluctuate at all?
- Have you been losing increasing amounts of weight?
- Has anything like this ever happened before?

Symptoms
- **Weight**
  - ➤ How much weight have you lost?
- **Appetite**
  - ➤ How has your appetite been?
- **Exercise**
  - ➤ How much have you been exercising? Is this normal for you?
- **Remember: "TIP ABCDE"**
  - ➤ **Tuberculosis** – Have you had a cough? Any night-sweats?
  - ➤ **Infection** – Have you been ill recently?
  - ➤ **Psychiatric** – How has your mood been? Felt particularly anxious?
  - ➤ **Addison's** – Have you felt tired? Any dizziness? Any change in skin colour?
  - ➤ **Bowels (IBD, Coeliac)** – How are your bowels/ stool? Any tummy pain?
  - ➤ **Cancer** – Any fevers?
  - ➤ **Diabetes** – Have you felt particularly thirsty? Passed more urine?
  - ➤ **Endocrine (Thyrotoxicosis)** – Have you felt hot? Tremor? Throat lump?
- General enquiry – other than the weight, have you noticed any other changes?

Systems
- **Consider asking about any system depending on what you have elicited so far. If you have no idea what is going on, try a quick bodily systems review:**
  - ➤ **Neurological** – Have you had a headache? Noticed a change in any of your senses? And what about any weakness or altered sensation?
  - ➤ **Cardiorespiratory** – Have you had any chest pain or discomfort? Any shortness-of-breath? Any coughing?
  - ➤ **Gastrointestinal** – Have you noticed any change in your bowels?
  - ➤ **Genitourinary** – And what about the waterworks?
  - ➤ **Gynaecological** – Is there any chance you could be pregnant?
  - ➤ **Musculoskeletal** – Have you noticed any joint or pain or stiffness?
  - ➤ **Psychiatric** – How has your mood been? Have you been feeling particularly anxious?
  - ➤ **Constitutional** – Have you felt tired? Fevers? Night-sweats?

ICE
- You've given me a lot of information, thank you. I'd like to hear a little about what you think could be going on. Do you have any idea?
- Is there anything that's particularly concerning you that you'd like to discuss?
- What exactly are you looking for today, resolution or reassurance?

PMHx
- Do you have any medical conditions?
- Ask a few specific questions to show that you're thinking about different causes
- Specifically, I'd like to ask if you've ever been diagnosed with:
    - Something called an autoimmune disease?
    - Bowel disease, diabetes, thyroid disease?
    - Have you ever been diagnosed with cancer?

DHx
- Are you on any medication? Anything over-the-counter or alternative medicines?
- Have any medications been changed recently?
- Are you allergic to anything that you know of?

SHx
- **S**moking/ Alcohol/ Recreational drugs
- **H**ome environment? Have you been getting support to cope with everything?
- **O**ccupation – What do you do for a living if you don't mind me asking? How has this impacted on your life and occupation?

Summarise and Thank
- I'd just like to summarise back to you to make sure I haven't missed anything
- Is there anything you'd like to talk about that we haven't quite addressed?
- Thank you for talking to me and I wish you all the best

Investigations

Examination	Full physical examination
Bedside	Urine dip, blood glucose
Bloods	FBC, studies, U&Es, LFTs, TFTs, tumour markers, HbA1c
Imaging	CXR, AXR, CT CAP
Special	Colonoscopy, endoscopy, short synacthen test, urea breath test

Top Tip! Tuberculosis affects pretty much every single body system and can therefore present in atypical ways. Always think Tuberculosis in someone with a positive travel history.

Differential Diagnosis

	Diagnosis	Features In History	Features In Investigations	Management
ENDOCRINE	**Hyperthyroidism**	Weight loss but increased appetite, associated with often young. palpitations (may be regular or irregular), sweats, diarrhoea, anxiety, irregular periods, heat intolerance.	Hand tremor, tachycardia, diaphoretic. ECG: sinus tachycardia or AF. TFTs: raised T4 suppressed TSH (in primary hyperthyroidism)	Commonly "Block and replace" with carbimazole and thyroxine in primary. Look for goitre, thyroid cancer and pituitary mass for secondary.
	Diabetes Mellitus	Polyuria, polydipsia, tiredness, weight loss, FH of DM, personal history of other autoimmune diseases.	Exam: may seem tired, dehydrated. Urine dip: glucose. Bloods: high glucose, HbA1c.	Rehydration, check for DKA and treat if present as emergency. T1DM: insulin T2DM: oral hypoglycaemics. Endocrinology referral.
	Addison's	Tiredness, weakness, poor appetite, weight loss, hyperpigmentation. Dizziness (orthostatic), myalgia (high-K$^+$) RF: history of other autoimmune diseases,	Exam: dehydration, hypotension (orthostatic). Bloods: low Na, high 9am cortisol, positive short synacthen test.	Steroid replacement therapy – urgent corticosteroids and IV NaCl in crisis. Endocrinology follow up.
GASTROINTESTINAL	**IBD**	Weight loss associated with frequent, intermittent, chronic, bloody/mucous loose stools, weight loss, anorexia, lethargy. Extra intestinal: eyes, joint pains, skin rashes, perianal abscess.	Generalised abdominal tenderness, may have RIF mass (ileocecal) Raised WCC, CRP. Faecal calprotectin raised. AXR may show thumb printing. Colonoscopy for biopsy	Rehydrate, Immunosuppression (prednisolone, azathioprine / 5-MP, infliximab etc. depending on response) to induce remission in acute flare.
	Coeliac Disease	Weight loss associated with history of steatorrhoea (oily, smelly, hard to flush), flatulence, lethargy. May have other autoimmune diseases/ FHx	Examination: abdomen may be distended. Bloods: electrolyte deficiencies, anaemia. Small bowel biopsy: anti-TTG and anti-gliadin antibodies.	Patient education and support. Gluten free diet.
	GORD	Reduced appetite / fear of eating due to burning central chest pain, worse lying down and leaning forward, worse after meals, obesity, may radiate towards neck	Normal ECG, CXR may show hiatus hernia. Positive urea breath test if *H. Pylori.*	PPI and simple antacids. Weight loss. Consider *H. pylori* as cause and eradicate.

	Diagnosis	Features In History	Features In Investigations	Management
RESPIRATORY	**Tuberculosis**	Weight loss associated with ongoing productive cough, fevers, appetite loss, night sweats. Travel to endemic TB region in last year, or previous TB, no BCG vaccine.	Apical reduced air entry and crackles. CXR: apical consolidation. Bloods: raised WCC, CRP, Quantiferon +ve. Early morning sputum positive for acid fast bacilli.	Commence anti-TB treatment (RIPE for 2 months then RI for 4 months). Contact precautions in hospital.
	Pulmonary Cachexia (COPD)	Weight loss over a long time associated with history of cough and shortness of breath on exertion or with precipitants. COPD – history of smoking (usually 20+ pack years), chest infections in the winter, "smokers cough".	Examination: reduced expansion, bilateral wheeze, tachypnoea, reduced saturations. Reduced peak flow. CXR: may see focus of infection. Hyper inflated lungs in COPD. Obstructive pattern on spirometry.	Education on control and optimisation of medication, maximise function and reduce work of breathing.
OTHER	**Cancer**	B-symptoms (FLAWS): fever, lethargy, appetite loss, weight loss, sweats. May be able to pin down organ with systems review.	Full examination of all systems. Urine dip and blood tests incl. Cancer markers (CEA, PSA, CA 125, CA 19-9, AFP)	Urgent 2WW for relevant specialty, counselling and MDT approach to treatment.
	Depression	Reduced appetite, tiredness, lack of interest in doing things, early morning waking, low mood. Screen thoughts of deliberate self-harm and suicide. May have history of mental illness, emotional trauma. Ask about risk factors.	Nil findings on physical examination or bloods – have to screen for organic causes. Signs of depression on MSE.	Bio-psycho-social approach with advice re: diet, hydration and exercise. Psychotherapy / CBT. Medication such as SSRIs.

Also Consider: Pool Oral intake due to mobility/social issues or Anorexia Nervosa

Marking Criteria WEIGHT/ APPETITE LOSS	Marks	
	Awarded	Available
Washed hands at the start of the station		1
Introduced themselves – Including First name, last name and role		1
Patient details confirmed: Full name, Age/ D.O.B.		1
Explained purpose of consultation		1
Open question about what brings the patient in today + Clarification of any ambiguity		1
Timeline allows a clear understanding of onset and progression - Onset/ Circumstance - Sudden vs. gradual - Fluctuations - Progression - Past episodes		3

Symptoms elicited are relevant and clearly directed at either arriving at a diagnosis or excluding other plausible diagnoses
- Weight
- Appetite
- Exercise
- **"TIP ABCDE"**
   o **Tuberculosis** – Have you had a cough? Any night-sweats?
   o **Infection** – Have you been ill recently?
   o **Psychiatric** – How has your mood been? Felt particularly anxious?
   o **Addison's** – Have you felt tired? Dizzy? Any change in skin colour?
   o **Bowels (IBD, Coeliac)** – How are your bowels/ stool? Any tummy pain?
   o **Cancer** – Any fevers?
   o **Diabetes** – Have you felt particularly thirsty? Passed more urine?
   o **Endocrine (Thyrotoxicosis)** – Have you felt hot? Tremor? Throat lump?
- General enquiry – other than the weight, have you noticed any other changes?
		5

Systems queried are relevant to the complaint and adequate questions are asked for each symptom - Neurological; Cardiorespiratory; Gastrointestinal; Genitourinary; Gynaecological; Musculoskeletal; Psychiatric; Constitutional		5
Explores **Ideas, Concerns and Expectations**		3
Elicits relevant **Past Medical History** - Autoimmunity; bowel disease; DM; thyroid problems; fibromyalgia; malignancy		2
Elicits relevant **Drug History** including **Allergies**		2
Elicits relevant **Family History**		2
Elicits relevant **Social History** – including Smoking/ alcohol/ recreational drugs; **Home** environment and support; **Occupation** and impact on life		2
Closes consultation appropriately allowing the patient to ask any questions		1
Presentation: structured, concise		2
Appropriate Differential Diagnosis ± Investigations ± Management Plan		3
Examiner mark – professionalism and rapport		5
Patient mark – professionalism and rapport		5

Consultation	Presentation	Global marks patient	Global marks examiner	Total
30	5	5	5	45

15F brought in by her mother as she is losing weight

HPC	Mother says her daughter has been losing weight rapidly over the past months, but thinks this is getting worse. Daughter is sitting quietly in the corner of the room. Daughter is avoiding eye contact and provides short answers. Says she just hasn't been feeling hungry. Does not want to eat because she does not like her mother's cooking. Says she has been exercising more than usually because she wants to get better at netball – her passion. She is adamant that she has been having a significant growth spurt. She denies any diarrhoea or vomiting. No abdominal pain. No Nausea. No headaches or SOB. Says she has stopped having her period some months ago.
PMHx	Pneumonia age 8, required ITU, Asthma.
DHx	Vitamins she buys online with friends
SHx	Lives at home with mother, parents divorced. Does not want to see father and his new wife anymore. Looks after her younger brother as mother works a lot. Dreams of a career as a model.
ICED	"I'm alright, there's nothing wrong with me. My mother is just overreacting"
Ix	FBC, U&E, LFT, TFT, LH, FSH, oestradiol, prolactin, vitamin B, folate, iron levels, ECG.
Dx	Anorexia Nervosa
Tx	Refer to CAMS for psychotherapy and community support. If high risk then Inpatient admission with NG feeding, electrolyte monitoring and regular ECGs.

85F referred by GP with weight loss

HPC	4 months history of weight loss. Lost 5 stone in last 4 months. Denies being on diet. Says she has been feeling somewhat more tired and feels like she is out of breath faster than she used to be. Has been feeling constipated for some time, but feels this is getting worse. Decreased appetite. Has been having a cough for a while. No haemoptysis. Denies CP, nausea or vomiting. No headaches. Reports small amounts of PR bleeding (fresh blood). She feels her abdomen is getting a bit distended and someone recently commented that her eyes look yellow.
PMHx	COPD, Asbestosis, uterine fibroids
DHx	Inhalers, bisoprolol, Aspirin.
SHx	Widowed. Used to work in a chemical plant. Smoked since aged 20. Currently smokes 20 cigarettes per day, used to smoke more. Drinks 1 bottle of wine per day.
ICED	"Did I give myself cancer Doctor?"
Ix	FBC, LFT, U&E, Vit B, CXR, consider CT chest abdomen and pelvis, occult faecal blood, biopsy of appropriate, Ascites aspiration for routine and histopathology
Dx	Mesothelioma (background of Asbestos exposure) with Ascites (peritoneal/liver metastases)
Tx	Oncology referral, chemotherapy and surgical therapy less likely in view of possible metastases, radiotherapy for symptom control. Palliative care and McMillan referral. Analgesia.

7M presents with parents for weight loss

HPC	6-months history of weight loss. He has been unwell some 8 months ago, recovered, and then started losing weight. He has been sleepier and less able to focus. He has been less energetic and school performance has dropped with teachers complaining that he does not participate as much anymore and takes lots of toilet breaks. Has started wetting the bed again. He is drinking more than he used to. He says that he used to play football but finds it hard to keep up now. Denies any abdominal pain, palpitations, chest pain or SOB. No nausea or vomiting.
PMHx	Nil. Vaccinations up to date.
DHx	Nil. NKDA
SHx	Lives with family. Both parents work in a bank, child at school most of the day. Neither smoke. Boy used to play football – too tired now.
FHx	Grandmother had diabetes diagnosed aged 11 years, died age 45 years.
ICED	"I just want to play football again with my friends."
Ix	BM, blood glucose, serum ketones, FBC, LFT, U&E, Hb1AC, antibodies (GAD, IA2 Antigen) Serum insulin, ABG (if acutely unwell to r/o DKA)
Dx	Type 1 Diabetes
Tx	Start Insulin, education to parents (glucose monitoring, sick day rules, hypoglycaemia identification), notify school (glucose testing, insulin administration, hypoglycaemia, exercise).

WEIGHT GAIN
GENERAL FRAMEWORK

"WIPE" – Introduce yourself, whilst gaining consent
- Wash hands
- Introduce self – "Hello, my name is X and I am a medical student"
- Patient details – "Could I ask your full name and age?"
- Explain – "I have been asked to speak with you about what brings you in, would that be alright?"

Open
- I understand you've gained some weight recently. Would you mind telling me a little about what's been going on?
- **Clarification**

Timeline
- When did you first start gaining weight? Did anything happen around then?
- Has the weight gain been sudden or gradual?
- Does your weight fluctuate at all?
- Have you been gaining increasing amounts of weight?
- Has anything like this ever happened before?

Symptoms
- **Weight**
  - ➢ How much weight have you gained?
- **Appetite**
- How has your appetite been?
- **Exercise**
  - ➢ How much have you been exercising? Is this normal for you?
- **Remember: "HHPPCCR"**
  - ➢ **Heart Failure** – have you felt breathless? Worse when you lie down? At night? Ankle and lower back swelling?
  - ➢ **Hypothyroidism** – Cold intolerance? Constipation? Infrequent periods?
  - ➢ **PCOS** – Infrequent periods? Increased body hair? Acne? Darkened skin?
  - ➢ **Pregnancy** – Sexually active? When was LMP?
  - ➢ **Cushing's** – Swollen face? Purple skin marks? Bruising? More body hair?
  - ➢ **Cirrhosis** – Swollen ankles/ lower back? Fluid in tummy?
  - ➢ **Renal failure** – Swollen ankles/ lower back? Fluid in tummy?

Systems
- **Consider asking about any system depending on what you have elicited so far. If you have no idea what is going on, try a quick bodily systems review:**
  - ➢ **Neurological** – Have you had a headache? Noticed a change in any of your senses? And what about any weakness or altered sensation?
  - ➢ **Cardiorespiratory** – Have you had any chest pain or discomfort? Any shortness-of-breath? Any coughing?
  - ➢ **Gastrointestinal** – Have you noticed any change in your bowels?
  - ➢ **Genitourinary** – And what about the waterworks?
  - ➢ **Gynaecological** – Is there any chance you could be pregnant?
  - ➢ **Musculoskeletal** – Have you noticed any joint or pain or stiffness?
  - ➢ **Psychiatric** – How has your mood been? Have you been feeling particularly anxious?
  - ➢ **Constitutional** – Have you felt tired? Fevers? Night-sweats?

ICE
- You've given me a lot of information, thank you. I'd like to hear a little about what you think could be going on. Do you have any idea?
- Is there anything that's particularly concerning you that you'd like to discuss?
- What exactly are you looking for today, resolution or reassurance?

PMHx
- Do you have any medical conditions?
- Ask a few specific questions to show that you're thinking about different causes
- Specifically, I'd like to ask if you've ever been diagnosed with:
    ➢ Heart problems? Thyroid problems? Polycystic ovaries? Hepatitis? Liver failure? Kidney failure?

DHx
- Are you on any medication? Anything over-the-counter or alternative medicines?
- Have any medications been changed recently?
- Are you allergic to anything that you know of?

FHx
- Do any conditions run in the family? Consider asking specifics as for PMHx!
- Has anyone in the family ever gone through anything similar to what you're going though?

SHx
- Smoking/ Alcohol/ Recreational drugs
- Home environment? Have you been getting support to cope with everything?
- Occupation – What do you do for a living if you don't mind me asking? How has this impacted on your life and occupation?

Summarise and Thank
- I'd just like to summarise back to you to make sure I haven't missed anything
- Is there anything you'd like to talk about that we haven't quite addressed?
- Thank you for talking to me and I wish you all the best

Investigations

Examination	Full examination including thyroid.
Bedside	Urine dip, blood glucose, postural blood pressure
Bloods	FBC, U&E, LFTs, CRP, ESR, TFTs
Imaging	CXR, USS abdomen
Special	24 hour cortisol, desmopressin suppression, liver screen, echocardiogram

Differential Diagnosis

	Diagnosis	Features In History	Features In Investigations	Management
ENDOCRINE	**Hypothyroidism**	Weight gain, Tiredness cold intolerance, constipation, irregular periods, dry skin and hair. FH or personal history of autoimmune diseases.	Full examination including thyroid exam – goitre, bradycardia, slowed reflexes, dry hair. Bloods: raised TSH, low or normal T4.	Thyroxine to treat and tirate to TSH. Consider other autoimmune diseases that may also be present.
	Cushing's	Weight gain, "moon face", interscapula fat pad, central obesity, striae, easy bruising, hirsutism, depression. Females: amenorrhoea, inferitility, decreased libido. Steroid use long term in Cushing's syndrome.	Signs of Cushing's on exam (see left). 9 am cortisol low. Dexmethasone supression test positive in Cushing's disease. Look for source of ectopic ACTH (tumour)	Gradual withdrawal of causative medication in syndrome. In endogenous causes, treat underlying cause.
	Obesity	Excessive eating and inadequate exercise, sedentary job, poor diet.	Increased BMI, no findings for Cushing's or other causes.	Lifestyle advice re: diet and exercise.
FLUID OVERLOAD	**Heart Failure**	Progressive weight gain (ankle swelling, abominal swelling), shortness of breath, orthopnoea, PND, cough of frothy pink sputum, no fever, ankle oedema, history of cardiac disease, cardiac risk factors (HTN, DM, FHx, smoking, lipids, obesity)	Reduced saturation, tachypnoea, bilateral crackles on examination / and dullness to percussion if effusion present, pitting oedema, S3 heart sound of volume overload. CXR: fluid overload Bloods: raised BNP Echo: reduced ejection fraction	Offload fluid with diuretics, monitor U&Es, disease modifying medications of heart failure and symptomatic relief (ACEi, spironolactone, beta blocker)
	Renal Failure	Progressive weight gain (ankle swelling, abominal swelling) with history of kidney disease (may be secondary to HTN, diabetes, PKD, glomerulonephritis)	Examination: evidence of fluid overload, may have ballotable kidneys (PKD) or signs of diabetes / HTN. Bloods: reduced eGFR, raised urea and creatinine	Offload fluid, monitor U&Es, referral to nephrologist ?need for dialysis.
	Ascites secondary to Liver Failure	Abdominal distension and weight gain. May have history of haematemesis, previous episodes of abdominal distension, pancreatitis. history of alcohol excess, hepatitis B/C.	Shifting dullness on abdominal examination, may have peripheral oedema also present. Bloods: abnormal LFTs (2:1 AST:ALT ratio in EtOH excess), raised GGT. Liver screen and USS liver.	Alcohol cessation. Treat complications of cirrhosis. Avoid hepatotoxins. Assess suitability for transplant with King's Criteria.

Also consider: Physiological causes e.g. Pregnancy

Marking Criteria WEIGHT GAIN	Marks	
	Awarded	Available
Washed hands at the start of the station		1
Introduced themselves – Including First name, last name and role		1
Patient details confirmed: Full name, Age/ D.O.B.		1
Explained purpose of consultation		1
Open question about what brings the patient in today + Clarification of any ambiguity		1
Timeline allows a clear understanding of onset and progression - Onset/ Circumstance - Sudden vs. gradual - Fluctuations - Progression - Past episodes		3

Symptoms elicited are relevant and clearly directed at either arriving at a diagnosis or excluding other plausible diagnoses
- Weight
- Appetite
- Exercise
- **"HHPPCCR"**
  o **Heart Failure** – have you felt breathless? Worse when you lie down? At night? Ankle and lower back swelling?
  o **Hypothyroidism** – Cold intolerance? Constipation? Infrequent periods?
  o **PCOS** – Infrequent periods? Increased body hair? Acne? Darkened skin?
  o **Pregnancy** – Sexually active? When was LMP?
  o **Cushing's** – Swollen face? Purple skin marks? Bruising? More body hair?
  o **Cirrhosis** – Swollen ankles/ lower back? Fluid in tummy?
  o **Renal failure** – Swollen ankles/ lower back? Fluid in tummy?
- General enquiry – other than the weight, have you noticed any other changes?
		5

Systems queried are relevant to the complaint and adequate questions are asked for each symptom - Neurological; Cardiorespiratory; Gastrointestinal; Genitourinary; Gynaecological; Musculoskeletal; Psychiatric; Constitutional		5
Explores **Ideas, Concerns and Expectations**		3
Elicits relevant **Past Medical History** - Heart problems; Thyroid problems; Polycystic ovaries; Hepatitis; Liver failure; Kidney failure		2
Elicits relevant **Drug History** including **Allergies**		2
Elicits relevant **Family History**		2
Elicits relevant **Social History** – including Smoking/ alcohol/ recreational drugs; **H**ome environment and support; **O**ccupation and impact on life		2
Closes consultation appropriately allowing the patient to ask any questions		1
Presentation: structured, concise		2
Appropriate Differential Diagnosis ± Investigations ± Management Plan		3
Examiner mark – professionalism and rapport		5
Patient mark – professionalism and rapport		5

Consultation	Presentation	Global marks patient	Global marks examiner	Total
‾‾ 30	‾ 5	‾ 5	‾ 5	‾ 45

60M, presenting with weight gain.

HPC	Weight gain for about 2 to 3 months despite trying to lose weight. He has particularly gained weight in his face and around his abdomen which is abnormal for him. He normally does not gain weight very easily. He has also noted that he bruises more easily than normally. He does not report to be eating more or exercising less. He has not changed his lifestyle either. He does not report nausea, vomiting or diarrhoea. No SOB or CP. He generally feels well, but reports feeling more sluggish recently and less motivated. He is struggling to keep up at work and finds he has a reduced concentration span.
PMHx	COPD, frequent chest infections.
SHx	Lives at home with wife. Has 3 children. Been smoking for 40 years. Has been diagnosed with COPD and has been given some new pills by his GP.
DHx	"Some new pills from my GP after I was getting lots of chest infections". Takes inhalers (blue and purple one) regularly. NKDA.
ICE	"I just want to lose the weight I have been gaining.
Dx	Corticosteroid associated weight gain
Ix	FBC, TFT, LFT, glucose, 24 hours urinary cortisol, overnight dexamethasone suppression test
Tx	Reduce dose of steroids. Consider prophylactic antibiotics and chest physiotherapy to improve respiratory function and prevent further chest infections.

50F presenting with weight gain and increasing fatigue.

HPC	She has been feeling more tired for some time now. She feels less motivated and finds it harder to get going in the morning. She is also lower in mood and she feel like she is colder than she normally is. She also finds that she has lowered libido. She also no longer enjoys walking her dog and exercising, both of which are things she used to love and do religiously some months back. She also spends less time with her friends because she finds it hard to motivate herself to go out. She feels sluggish and sleeps more than she used to. No nausea, vomiting or diarrhoea. She does not report change in exercise level, but does feel less motivated to move and more tired than usually. She is getting more constipated. She has gone through menopause without any problems.
PMHx	Nil relevant. 2 children delivered via C-section.
SHx	Separated, lives alone. Works in bank.
DHx	HRT, Gaviscon.
ICE	"I just wants to understand why I'm gaining weight and why I feel so tired and cold all the time."
Dx	Hypothyroidism.
Ix	FBC, TFT, LFTs, U&Es, thyroid USG, antibodies (thyroid peroxidase, thyroid receptor).
Tx	Thyroxine according to individual requirements

29F presenting with weight gain and increasing fatigue.

HPC	She has been feeling more tired for some time now. She feels less motivated and finds it harder to get going in the morning. She is also lower in mood and she feel like she is colder than she normally is. She also finds that she has lowered libido. She also no longer enjoys walking her dog and exercising, both of which are things she used to love and do religiously some months back. No nausea, vomiting or diarrhoea. She does not report change in exercise level, but does feel less motivated to move and more tired than usually. She is getting more constipated. She has gone through menopause without any problems. She delivered a child by Caesarean section and required blood transfusion, post operatively, due to heavy bleeding. She was unable to breast feed and has not resumed her periods since.
PMHx	Nil relevant. 1 children delivered via C-section 18 months ago.
SHx	Married, Works in an opera house as production manager.
DHx	Gaviscon.
ICE	"I just wants to understand why I'm gaining weight and why I feel so tired and cold all the time."
Dx	Hypothyroidism as result of Sheehan's syndrome. Other possibility is growth hormone deficiency
Ix	FBC, TFT, LFTs, U&Es, prolactin, cortisol (short synacthen test is ideal to detect cortisol deficiency) ACTH, (LH FSH, IGF-1, antibodies (thyroid peroxidase, thyroid receptor), thyroid USG, MRI Pituitary.
Tx	Thyroxine, may require other hormone replacement e.g. hydrocortisone for secondary steroid deficiency

65M presenting to his GP with weight gain.

HPC	He has been observing a gradual weight gain. This has been getting much worse over the last few weeks. He also noticed that he feels increasingly short of breath and finds it more and more difficult to walk long distances as he gets painful calves and feels like his chest is constricted by a heavy band. He has also noticed swelling in his lower legs. This gets worse as day progresses. He has noted some SOB, but no palpitations. No sweating, nausea or vomiting. No fever or cough. He finds himself more tired at the end of the day which he ascribes to the increased work in breathing and the generally increased effort of getting around.
PMHx	Triple bypass surgery, Angina, Tablet controlled diabetes.
DHx	Bisoprolol, Aspirin, GTN, metformin
SHx	Ex-smoker. Obese, BMI of 34. Lives at home, alone.
ICE	"I'm worried that all the weight gain is due to my diabetes being poorly controlled."
Dx	Heart failure with peripheral oedema.
Ix	FBC, U&Es, Troponin, BNP, ECG, CXR, Trans-thoracic echo.
Tx	Treat fluid overload with diuretics such as furosemide or spironolactone. Ensure to monitor weight and renal function, in particular Creatinine and potassium.

FEVERS & NIGHT SWEATS
GENERAL FRAMEWORK

<u>**"WIPE"**</u> – Introduce yourself, whilst gaining consent
- Wash hands
- Introduce self – "Hello, my name is X and I am a medical student"
- Patient details – "Could I ask your full name and age?"
- Explain – "I have been asked to speak with you about what brings you in, would that be alright?"

<u>**Open**</u>
- I understand you've had a fever recently. Would you mind telling me a little about what's been going on?
- **Clarification** – When you say feverish, do you mean you feel hot or cold?

<u>**Timeline**</u>
1. When did you first notice the fever? Did anything happen around then?
2. Did the fever come on suddenly or gradually?
3. Does it come and go or is it there all the time?
4. Has it been getting progressively worse?
5. Have you had it before?

<u>**Symptoms**</u>
- Have you taken a temperature?
- Have you been sweating a lot? More at night?

Is it alright if I ask you some general screening questions to try and understand what could be going on? (Jump straight into the review of bodily systems...)

<u>**Systems**</u> – Remember as **head to toe**!
- **Neurological** – Have you had a headache? Noticed a change in any of your senses? And what about any weakness or altered sensation?
  - ➤ Think **meningitis** – ask about: headache/ stiff neck/ worse with light/ rash
  - ➤ Think **temporal arteritis** – ask about loss of vision/ pain on chewing/ tender sides of the head
- **Cardiorespiratory** – Have you had any chest pain or discomfort? Any shortness-of-breath? Any coughing?
  - ➤ Think **chest infection** – ask about chest pain worse on breathing in/ SOB/ coughing ± sputum/ blood
- **Gastrointestinal** – Have you noticed any change in your bowels? Any tummy pain or discomfort?
  - ➤ Think **IBD/ cancer, etc**. – ask about vomiting/ diarrhoea/ tummy pain/ PR bleed
  - ➤ Think **hepatitis** – Viral illness? Noticed any yellowing of skin?
- **Genitourinary** – And what about the waterworks?
  - ➤ Think **UTI**, potential pyelonephritis – ask frequency/ urgency/ stinging pain on urination
- **Gynaecological** – Is there any chance you could be pregnant?
  - ➤ Think **ectopic pregnancy** – ask if sexually active/ last menstrual period
- **Musculoskeletal** – Have you noticed any joint or muscle pain or stiffness?
  - ➤ Think **connective tissue disease** (E.g. SLE) or **RA** – ask about morning stiffness, small joints are hot and tender
- **Constitutional** – Have you felt tired? Any loss of appetite? Any weight loss?
  - ➤ Think **malignancy** – ask questions specific to suspected malignancy – E.g. Haemoptysis, PR bleed, breast lump, bruising/ anaemia/ infections (*haematological* malignancy)
- **Dermatological** – Any skin changes? Rashes? Ulcers? (Consider vasculitis, connective tissue disease, etc.)

- **+ ENQUIRE ABOUT RECENT TRAVEL**
  - ➢ DVT = swollen leg? Recent long-haul flight?
  - ➢ Malaria/ Typhoid/ HIV = recent travel to endemic area + fever!
  - ➢ TB = weight loss, night-sweats, travel to/ contact with person from endemic area

- **+ ENQUIRE ABOUT SEXUAL CONTACT**
  - ➢ EBV (Mononucleosis) – university fresher, exchanged saliva through kissing/ sharing cups – Noticed neck lumps? Had a sore throat? Felt ill?
  - ➢ Sexually transmitted infection – any recent unprotected sexual contact (including oral/ vaginal/ anal)?

ICE
- You've given me a lot of information, thank you. I'd like to hear a little about what you think could be going on. Do you have any idea?
- Is there anything that's particularly concerning you that you'd like to discuss?
- What exactly are you looking for today, resolution or reassurance?

PMHx
- Do you have any medical conditions?
- Ask a few specific questions to show that you're thinking about different causes
- Specifically, I'd like to ask if you've ever been diagnosed with:
  - ➢ Rheumatoid arthritis/ Cancer/ STIs/ UTIs

DHx
- On any medication? Any doses of medication changed?
- Any allergies?

FHx
- Any conditions run in the family?
  - ➢ Autoimmune disease; diabetes; cancer; thyroid disease
  - ➢ Do any friends/ family have any infections at the moment?

SHx –
- Smoking/ Alcohol/ Recreational drugs
- Home environment? Support?
- Occupation – impact on life and on occupation?

Summarise and Thank
- I'd just like to summarise back to you to make sure I haven't missed anything
- Is there anything you'd like to talk about that we haven't quite addressed?
- Thank you for talking to me and I wish you all the best

Investigations

Examination	Full examination, including lymphadenopathy and ENT
Bedside	Temperature, swabs, urine dip
Bloods	FBC, U&E, CRP, ESR, thick and thin films, HIV test, autoimmune screen, LDH, quantiferon, blood cultures (on all febrile patients)
Imaging	CXR, USS abdo, ?CT head if neuro symptoms
Special	Echocardiogram, bone marrow biopsy, urine MC&S

Differential Diagnosis

	Diagnosis	Features In History	Features In Investigations	Management
INFECTIVE	**Meningitis**	Prodromal illness, fever, neck stiffness, rash, photophobia	Kernig's positive on examination, non-blanching rash, raised WCC and CRP	Admit to hospital. Immediate antibiotics
	Tuberculosis	Weight loss associated with ongoing productive cough, fevers, appetite loss, night sweats. Travel to endemic TB region in last year, or previous TB, no BCG vaccine.	Apical reduced air entry and crackles. CXR: apical consolidation. Bloods: raised WCC, CRP, Quantiferon +ve. Early morning sputum positive for acid fast bacilli.	Commence anti-TB treatment (RIPE for 2 months then RI for 4 months). Contact precautions in hospital.
	Malaria	Fever in a returning traveller from endemic region (classically cyclical 24-48h). Fatigue, rigors, arthralgia. May have abdominal pain, neurological symptoms (*P. Falciparum* – poorer prognosis). Ask about anti-malarial prophylaxis, bites, use of anti-insect devices (nets / sprays).	Exam: no specific findings; mosquito bites, generalised abdominal tenderness. Bloods: Classic triad: thrombocytopenia, elevated LDH levels, and atypical lymphocytes. Thick and thin films for parasitic load and typing.	Anti-malarials depending on guidelines of type and area of world. Generally, Artesunate, or quinine if unavailable.
	Infective Endocarditis	Ongoing fever, malaise, chest pain, SOB, anorexia, weight loss, clubbing of fingers. No URTI/ Resp / Abdo symptoms. RF: IVDU, dental procedures without antibiotic cover, gingivitis, previous valve disease/ replacement.	Exam: new murmur, Janeway lesions, Osler's nodes, splinter haemorrhages, Roth spots. Urine: proteinuria, microscopic haematuria Bloods: may see low Hb. Raised WCC. Positive blood cultures (need 3 sets). Echo: valvular vegetations. Calculate Duke's criteria.	Aggressive, prolonged, multiple antibiotic therapy depending on culture results (common: penicillin, ceftriaxone, gentamicin)
	HIV Seroconversion	Fever, malaise, tiredness, myalgia, rash; roughly 4-6 weeks after high risk exposure (MSM, visit to endemic area with unprotected sexual encounters, IVDU sharing needles)	Exam: no viral source found, lymphadenopathy. Serological tests for HIV. Bloods including CD4+ count and viral load following diagnosis.	Specialist HIV follow up and highly active anti-retroviral therapy and screening for associated infections and problems (TB, lipids, colon cancer etc.).

	Diagnosis	Features In History	Features In Investigations	Management
NON - INFECTIVE	**Lymphoma / leukaemia**	B-symptoms (FLAWS): fever, lethargy, appetite loss, weight loss, sweats. Fever may be cyclical in nature (Pel-Ebstein). May have noted swollen lymph nodes in neck, axilla, groin.	Full examination of all systems including lymph nodes in neck, axilla and groin. Urine dip and blood tests. Bloods: extremely raised WCC. Bone marrow / lymph node biopsy shows dysmorphic cells.	Urgent 2WW, counselling and MDT approach to treatment.
	Vasculitis	Fevers, malaise, weight loss, fatigue. Systemic symptoms: skin (nodules / rash / Raynaud's / ulcers), respiratory (rhinitis, polyps, chronic cough, haemoptysis), MSk (myalgia / arthritis), neuro (headache / seizure / focal neurological signs). May be post viral.	Exam: 4 limb BPs may show difference / saddle nose, lymphadenopathy / decreased breath sounds, wheeze / abnormal heart sounds / hepato/spleno-megaly / rash, swollen joints. Bloods: Raised ESR, CRP, p-/ c-ANCA, lupus anticoagulant, beta-2 microglobulin, anti-CCP, ANA. CT chest if chest symptoms may show ground glass.	Immunosuppression is mainstay of treatment.
	Menopause	Night sweats and hot flushes during the day without triggers. Other symptoms may be: poor sleep, decreased cognition and memory, erratic mood,	Nil findings on examination. Bloods: peri-menopausal levels of LH and FSH (both high, FSH>LH)	Education and support, symptomatic management. HRT for intolerable symptoms.

Also consider:

- Osteomyelitis if there are open wounds
- Intra-abdominal Collections E.g. Post-Surgery or with Pancreatitis
- Other tropical diseases e.g. Dengue Fever
- Atypical presentations: nocturnal hypoglycaemia (pre-bed insulin), alcohol withdrawal

Marking Criteria FEVERS/ NIGHT SWEATS	Marks	
	Awarded	Available
Washed hands at the start of the station		1
Introduced themselves – Including First name, last name and role		1
Patient details confirmed: Full name, Age/ D.O.B.		1
Explained purpose of consultation		1
Open question about what brings the patient in today + Clarification of any ambiguity		1
Timeline allows a clear understanding of onset and progression - Onset/ Circumstance - Sudden vs. gradual - Fluctuations - Progression - Past episodes		3
Symptoms elicited are relevant and clearly directed at either arriving at a diagnosis or excluding other plausible diagnoses - Temperature? - Sweating? Especially at night? - General enquiry – other than the fever, have you noticed any other changes?		5
Systems queried are relevant to the complaint and adequate questions are asked for each symptom - Neurological; Cardiorespiratory; Gastrointestinal; Genitourinary; Gynaecological; Musculoskeletal; Dermatological; Psychiatric; Constitutional; **RECENT TRAVEL; SEXUAL CONTACT**		5
Explores **Ideas, Concerns and Expectations**		3
Elicits relevant **Past Medical History** - RA; Cancer; STIs; UTIs		2
Elicits relevant **Drug History** including **Allergies**		2
Elicits relevant **Family History**		2
Elicits relevant **Social History** – including Smoking/ alcohol/ recreational drugs; **H**ome environment and support; **O**ccupation and impact on life		2
Closes consultation appropriately allowing the patient to ask any questions		1
Presentation: structured, concise		2
Appropriate Differential Diagnosis ± Investigations ± Management Plan		3
Examiner mark – professionalism and rapport		5
Patient mark – professionalism and rapport		5

Consultation	Presentation	Global marks patient	Global marks examiner	Total
‾30	‾5	‾5	‾5	‾45

25F student presents with a 3-week history of night sweats

HPC	Patient has been having night sweats and fever over night for the last 3 weeks. She has also been having a cough and has been feeling generally unwell. She has recently returned from a trip to Sri Lanka and Pakistan where she spent some time in the country side. She has been in a long-term relationship for the last 5 years. She feels she has lost weight (her clothes are loose). She reports no chest pain, no abdominal pain, no weight loss, no rashes. She stresses that she took all precautions of washing her hands and even prophylactic malaria treatment when on her trip.
PMHx	1 termination of pregnancy when she was 17
DHx	NKDA, on depot injection for contraception, takes Prozac occasionally.
SHx	Smokes cannabis & shisha on occasion, no IVDU. Long term relationship. Lives with boyfriend.
ICE	"I'm worried that my boyfriend might be cheating on me and has given me an STI."
Dx	Tuberculosis
Ix	FBC, CRP, LFT, U&Es, CXR, sputum for AFB, at least 3 sputum cultures (spontaneous or induced)
Tx	Involve Infectious Diseases team. Refer to CDC. Depending on strain, treat with Rifampicin, Isoniazid, pyrazinamide and ethambutol. Also need Pyridoxine

50M with night sweats and weight loss

HPC	Patient has been having night sweats and fevers for roughly 4 weeks. He has also noticed some weight loss and feels like he is getting sick more often than he used to. He has also noticed small non-painful swellings in his axillae. He feels more tired than usual. His bowels are normal and denies any recent changes. He has no joint pain/swellings nor rash. He reports no SOB, chest pain, infective symptoms (currently). No nausea, vomiting or diarrhoea. He had unprotected sex with a sex worker whilst on holiday in Bangkok 3 months ago.
PMHx	Glandular fever as a teenager, Hypertension – well controlled. Varicose veins, glandular fever, genital herpes.
DHx	Bisoprolol 2.5mg, Multivitamin.
SHx	Works in factory. Single. Non-smoker. Drinks socially, but not on regular basis. Homosexual
ICE	"Doctor, I'm concerned that I have HIV."
Dx	Hodgkins Lymphoma
Ix	FBC, U&E, LFTs, Blood film, HIV test, CXR, PET/CT scan of the chest, abdomen and pelvis, FNAC/excision biopsy of the lymph node
Tx	Refer to Oncology. Depends on stage of disease. Consider treatment with radiotherapy if isolated lymph node affected. Chemotherapy offers more wide-spread action. Consider bone marrow transplant as attempt for cure.

25M patient with high fevers for 3 days.

HPC	Patient presents to hospital with a history of 3 days of high fever. He has also been complaining of headaches and vomiting. He has significant pain in his joints and muscles. He has been on holiday in the pacific and returned 2 weeks ago. He also has significant reddening of the skin, resembling a sunburn. The patient recalls having travelled through wooded areas and slept under the open sky one night. He does not remember having been bitten by any insects, but does recall that there were mosquitoes around the campfire at night. He reports no nausea, vomiting or diarrhoea. Some SOB and coughing, but pretty much settled. Feels more irritable than usually. He took full vaccinations prior to travel but was not able to take the tablets as prescribed as they gave him hallucinations and made him depressed.
PMHx	Acid reflux, otherwise fit and well
DHx	Gaviscon
SHx	Works as a journalist and writes for outdoor journals. Travels a lot. Single.
ICE	"I'm concerned that I have malaria or HIV as I did not take my prophylaxis medication."
Dx	Dengue fever
Ix	FBC, U&E, LFT, CXR, viral PCR, blood cultures
Tx	Symptomatic and supportive.

LUMPS
"WOC SOCRATES"

"WIPE" – Introduce yourself, whilst gaining consent
- Wash hands
- Introduce self – "Hello, my name is X and I am a medical student"
- Patient details – "Could I ask your full name and age?"
- Explain – "I have been asked to speak with you about what brings you in, would that be alright?"

Open
- I understand you've come in with a lump? Would you like to tell me about it?
- **Clarification** – if anything is unclear

Site
- Where exactly is the lump?

Onset
1. When did you first notice the lump? Did anything happen around then?
2. Do you know if the lump appeared suddenly or gradually?
3. Does the lump come and go or is it always there?
4. Has it been getting larger?
5. Have you had it before?

Character (**Ask the questions you deem relevant from the mnemonic below**)
- **Shape** – What shape is it?
- **Colour** – Is it the same colour as the surrounding skin?
- **Consistency** – Is it hard or soft?
- **Tenderness** – Is it tender?
- **Temperature** – Is it hot?
- **Fixity** – Is it fixed to the body underneath?

Radiation
- Have you noticed any other lumps?

Associated symptoms
- Together with "Character" – ask any further questions about the lump
- Consider brief **systems** review to rule out any serious pathology
- If thyroid lump – be sure to ask about THYROID SYMPTOMS
  - ➤ **Thyroid** – Have you been especially intolerant of heat? Have you lost any weight? How have your bowels been? Have you noticed a tremor? Have you felt anxious? More personal question. How have your periods been?

Timing – done above

Exacerbating/ Relieving
- Does anything make the lump better?
- Does anything make it worse?
- E.g.: straining/ coughing/ changing position/ pushing it inside (reducing lump)/ hot or cold

Severity
- How badly is the lump impacting on your life?

ICE
- You've given me a lot of information, thank you. I'd like to hear a little about what you think could be going on. Do you have any idea?
- Is there anything that's particularly concerning you that you'd like to discuss?
- What exactly are you looking for today, resolution or reassurance?

PMHx
- Do you have any medical conditions?
- Ask a few specific questions to show that you're thinking about different causes:
- Specifically, I'd like to ask if you've ever been diagnosed with:
    - Thyroid problems? A hernia? Arthritis? (Ask if relevant depending on site)

DHx
- Are you on any medication? Anything over-the-counter or alternative medicines?
- Have any medications been changed recently?
- Are you allergic to anything that you know of?

FHx
- Do any conditions run in the family? Consider asking specifics as for PMHx!
- Has anyone in the family ever any lumps similar to the ones you have?

SHx
- Smoking/ Alcohol/ Recreational drugs
- Home environment? (If patient is worried) Have you been getting support to cope with everything?
- Occupation – What do you do for a living if you don't mind me asking? How has this impacted on your life and occupation?

Summarise and Thank
- I'd just like to summarise back to you to make sure I haven't missed anything
- Is there anything you'd like to talk about that we haven't quite addressed?
- Thank you for talking to me and I wish you all the best

Investigations

Examination	Lump examination, lymph nodes, system exam / ENT if indicated
Bloods	FBC, U&E, CRP, tumour markers, TFTs
Imaging	USS lump, CT CAP if suspicious of cancer
Special	Lump fine needle aspiration / biopsy, mammogram

Differential Diagnosis

	Diagnosis	Features In History	Features In Investigations	Management
ABDOMINAL LUMP	**Lymph Nodes**	Lump: round, smooth, may be tender. Ass. With concurrent or recent infection. May be in neck, groin or axillae, and have other nodes too. Ask about B-symptoms (lymphoma) and systems review for infection source.	Exam: lymphadenopathy – check for splenomegaly and systemic upset. Bloods: raised WCC, CRP.	Depends on cause found – if infection reassure and treat. If red flags present for full work up and referral as appropriate.
	Hernia	Generally, groin or abdominal lump that is most prominent on straining, goes back in with relaxation or manipulation. Soft and variable in size. Ask about tenderness, red, hot, constipation, irreducibility, symptoms of obstruction.	Hernia exam – assess lump, signs of incarceration and strangulated hernia. USS to confirm hernia.	Watch and wait with conservative measures (trusses) if small. Surgical opinion for repair if worrying features.
THYOID LUMP	**Thyroglossal Cyst**	Neck lump, midline, usually asymptomatic. Ask about complications: dysphagia, obstructed breathing, infection (warm, painful, lymph nodes), fistula (skin opening with fluid)	Exam: thyroid exam – small, mid line, moves with tongue protrusion. Bloods: nil USS to confirm diagnosis if no complications.	Only needs to be removed (surgical) if complications present e.g. infected cyst, thyroglossal fistula or carcinoma.
	Graves Disease	Diffuse neck swelling, may be tender and preceded by viral infection. Often young. Palpitations (may be regular or irregular), sweats, weight loss, diarrhoea, anxiety, increased appetite, irregular periods, heat intolerance. Ask about eye complications (corneal ulcers, subluxation etc.)	Examination: Hand tremor, tachycardia, generalised goitre (?tender), exophthalmos, proptosis and lid lag. ECG: sinus tachycardia or AF. Bloods: raised T4 low TSH, TRAb positive. Diffuse uptake on radionucleotide testing.	Commonly "Block and replace" with carbimazole and thyroxine in primary hyperthyroidism. Radioiodine may be used to induce remission (not in those with Graves' orbitopathy). Management of ophthalmic complications (usually surgical)
	Thyroid Cancer	Single unilateral lump, perhaps lymph nodes also Thyroid symptoms: weight loss, increased appetite, tremor, palpitations, anxiety if hot adenoma.	Examination: single lump, lymphadenopathy Adenoma would be solitary, may be tender. Hot uptake on radionucleotide scan.	Referral for 2WW if red flags present. Surgical resection is likely treatment with replacement therapy after.

	Diagnosis	Features In History	Features In Investigations	Management
	Lipoma	Lump, varying size (1cm to >10cm), soft, non-tender, no skin changes, may be multiple, history of similar lumps /family history. No systemic symptoms.	Examination: lump, regular shape and edges, soft, non-fluctuant, non-pulsatile, mobile, subcutaneous, not tethered to skin or muscle. USS: lipoma.	No intervention needed unless causing complications (ulceration) – then surgical removal.
	Sebaceous Cyst	Lump, usually <5cm, sometimes dischares pus, may be smelly. Commonly face/ scalp / neck / trunk.	Lump – regular shape (round), central punctum that may be discharging, may be hard and tender or asymptomatic.	Usually no treatment unless appears infected – then oral antibiotics.
BREAST LUMP	**Cancer**	Lump found, unilateral, hard, irregular. May be associated with lethargy, weight loss, anorexia. RF: family history, early menarche, hormonal therapy.	Breast examination – hard, irregular lump, peau d'orange, lymphadenopathy, spinal tenderness (mets). Bloods: raised CA 15-3 CT CAP for staging. Lymph node biopsy.	MDT approach with assessment for ?surgical resection, chemotherapy if known to be chemoresponsive (HER2)
	Fibroadenoma	Single, round, smooth, mobile, non-tender, unilateral lump. No systemic symptoms.	Single round, un tethered lump, no skin changes, may be tender. No lymphadenopathy. Bloods normal Diagnose on USS or FNA.	Reassure as it usually self resolves. *Always* safety net and encourage self-monitoring.
	Fibrocystic Change	Cyclical, tender, nodularity in breasts in line with menstrual cycle, no skin changes or systemic symptoms.	Generalised nodular feeling breasts, no skin changes, no spinal tenderness, resolves in different part of cycle.	Reassurance. *Always* safety net and encourage self-monitoring.
	Mastitis	Red, hot, tender lump with fevers in breastfeeding mothers with difficulties feeding. Usually unilateral.	Examination: red, raised lump in breast, hot, tender, indurated. (May be fluctuant if abscess present) Bloods: raised WCC	Encourage to keep emptying breast (feeding / pump), oral antibiotics (safe in breastfeeding).
	Fat Necrosis	May have history of trauma or breast surgery. More common in middle aged women with large breasts.	Examination: lump, may be poorly circumscribed, no skin changes, may be fluctuant. Mammogram and USS for diagnosis.	Reassurance and symptom relief if painful. *Always* safety net and encourage self-monitoring.

Marking Criteria LUMPS	Marks	
	Awarded	Available
Washes hands at the start of the station		1
Introduces themselves – Including First name, last name and role		1
Patient details confirmed: Full name, Age/ D.O.B.		1
Explains purpose of consultation		1
Open question about what brings the patient in today + Clarification of any ambiguity		1
Site – Enquires about exact location of lump		1
Onset (Timeline) – Asks questions to provide a clear understanding of onset and progression - Onset/ Circumstance - Sudden vs. gradual - Fluctuations - Progression - Past episodes		3
Character - Obtains an accurate description of the lump - Mnemonic: She Cuts The Fish PERfectly or SCCTTF		1
Radiation - Asks about lumps anywhere else		1
Associated symptoms - **Symptoms** elicited are relevant and clearly directed at either arriving at a diagnosis or excluding other plausible diagnoses - Any further questions about lump - **Systems** queried are relevant to the complaint and adequate questions are asked for each symptom - Any relevant systems; consider full systems review to rule out any pathology - If thyroid lump – be sure to ask about **THYROID SYMPTOMS** - Rule out malignancy by asking about **constitutional symptoms**		6
Timing - This has been done		0
Exacerbation/ Relief - Clearly asks if the patient has noticed any relieving/ exacerbating factors, providing appropriate examples if prompted (Ex. strain, cough, position, reducing, hot/ cold, etc.)		1
Severity - Subjective quantitative assessment of chest pain severity		1
Explores **Ideas, Concerns and Expectations**		3
Elicits relevant **Past Medical History** - Thyroid problems; Hernias; Arthritis		2
Elicits relevant **Drug History** including **Allergies**		2
Elicits relevant **Family History**		2
Elicits relevant **Social History** – including Smoking/ alcohol/ recreational drugs; **Home** environment and support; **Occupation** and impact on life		2
Closes consultation appropriately allowing the patient to ask any questions		1
Presentation: structured, concise		2
Appropriate Differential Diagnosis ± Investigations ± Management Plan		3
Examiner mark – professionalism and rapport		5
Patient mark – professionalism and rapport		5

Consultation	Presentation	Global marks patient	Global marks examiner	Total
30	5	5	5	45

50F patient presents with swelling in her neck

HPC	She notice a pea sized swelling in her neck that has been there for months, but now noticed an increase in the size. Not painful or uncomfortable. Does not cause any problems swallowing or breathing. Mainly cosmetic concern. She feels intermittent palpitations and has noticed weight loss. She thinks she is nervous all the time as she has shaky hands. Also feels like she is less able to deal with heat. She has not noticed any SOB, CP noisy breathing nor dizziness. Does not report increased frequency of infections. No coughs or colds, no vomiting, nausea or diarrhoea. Her sister has recently been diagnosed with breast cancer.
PMHx	Type 1 Diabetes
DHx	Insulin, paracetamol, occasional ibuprofen.
SHx	Office worker, independent in activities of daily life.
ICE	"I'm worried that I have cancer."
Dx	Goitre with thyrotoxicosis
Ix	TFT, FBC, USS neck/thyroid, Anti thyroid antibodies (Thyroid peroxidase and/or thyroid receptor)
Tx	Anti-thyroid medications such as Carbimazole or propylthiouracil. Other options are Radioactive iodine (RAI) therapy and/or surgery. RAI may lead to hypothyroidism requiring levothyroxine treatment for life. Surgical removal is an option if the goitre is large or RAI fails.

25F with breast lump

HPC	Patient presenting with 3-weeks history of painless rounded lemon sized lump in her breast. She found the lump when showering. She denies any pain in breast or nipple. Lump is not tender or inflamed. No changes in skin. Patient reports no bruising or trauma to the breast that she can remember. No discharge from lump itself or from nipple. No diabetes, no obesity. There is no fever, weight loss or night sweats. No systemic symptoms of infection or degeneration. Patient reports no SOB, CP, dizziness, cough or colds. No nausea, vomiting or diarrhoea. No trauma.
PMHx	Nil.
DHx	Oral contraceptive pill.
SHx	Student, plays rugby.
FHx	None relevant.
ICE	"I'm worried that I have an aggressive breast cancer. Will I have to have my breast removed?"
Dx	Benign lipoma, breast cyst or aggressive cancer. Unlikely to be at fat necrosis given large size.
Ix	FBC,USS or mammogram, consider hormonal scree followed by FNAC or biopsy
Tx	Excision or drainage. Advise patient that drained cysts may return requiring further surgery.

45M patient with lump on calf

HPC	Patient presents with a 3-weeks history of a painful lump on his right calf. He does not remember when the lump came up. Lump has been present for some time, but became painful 1.5 weeks ago. He does not report feeling systemically unwell. He has been feeling a little run down and finding it more difficult to focus. He does not report any fevers or weight loss. Does not remember any trauma or insect bites. Reports no headaches, dizziness, visual disturbances, nausea or vomiting. He is normally fit and well. No diabetes, no HTN, not obese. He says that the lump is red, swollen and warm. He finds that it's very painful to touch. He reports having scratched at the lump in the past because it was itchy, not itchy anymore.
PMHx	Had alcohol detox 10 years ago.
DHx	NKDA
SHx	Works as a gardener, mainly in public parks and woods.
FHx	Father diagnosed with skin cancer age 50.
ICE	"I'm worried I have cancer"
Dx	FBC, U&E, LFT.
Ix	Skin Abscess
Tx	Incision drainage of abscess with additional empirical antibiotics. Take swab of pus and send to lab for more targeted therapy when organisms are identified. Most likely to be skin commensals. Likely option of treatment is flucloxacillin. Orally or IV depending on how unwell the patient is.

JAUNDICE
GENERAL FRAMEWORK

"WIPE" – Introduce yourself, whilst gaining consent
- Wash hands
- Introduce self – "Hello, my name is X and I am a medical student"
- Patient details – "Could I ask your full name and age?"
- Explain – "I have been asked to speak with you about what brings you in, would that be alright?"

Open
- I understand you've noticed a yellowing of your skin/eyes. Would you mind telling me more about that?
- Clarification

Timeline
1. When did you first notice yellowing? Was anything else happening around then?
2. Did yellowing come on suddenly or gradually?
3. Does it come and go or is it there all the time?
4. Has it been getting progressively worse?
5. Have you ever had anything like this before?

Symptoms
- Itching – often associated with increased bilirubin
- Confusion – associated with liver failure/ Wilson's
- Recent viral illness – associated with enzyme deficiency – Gilbert's disease
- General enquiry – other than the yellowing, have you noticed any other changes?

Systems
- **Gastrointestinal** – Loss of appetite? Any vomiting? Tummy pain (Esp. RUQ)? Pale stools?
- **Genitourinary** – How have the waterworks been? Dark urine?
- **Constitutional** – Loss of appetite? Loss of weight? Tired? Fever?
- **+ ENQUIRE ABOUT RECENT TRAVEL**
  - ➤ DVT = swollen leg? Recent long-haul flight?
  - ➤ Malaria/ Typhoid/ HIV = recent travel to endemic area + fever!
  - ➤ TB = weight loss, night-sweats, travel to/ contact with person from endemic area
- **+ ENQUIRE ABOUT SEXUAL CONTACT**
  - ➤ EBV (Mononucleosis) can cause a mild Jaundice – university fresher, exchanged saliva through kissing/ sharing cups – Noticed neck lumps? Had a sore throat? Felt ill?
  - ➤ Sexually transmitted infection such as Hepatitis– any recent unprotected sexual contact (including oral/ vaginal/ anal)?

ICE
- You've given me a lot of information, thank you. I'd like to hear a little about what you think could be going on. Do you have any idea?
- Is there anything that's particularly concerning you that you'd like to discuss?
- What exactly are you looking for today, resolution or reassurance?

PMHx
- Do you have any medical conditions?
- Ask a few specific questions to show that you're thinking about different causes:
- Specifically, I'd like to ask if you've ever been diagnosed with:
  - ➤ Something called an autoimmune disease?
  - ➤ Gallstones? Hepatitis? Cirrhosis?
  - ➤ Have you ever been diagnosed with cancer?

DHx

- Are you on any medication? Anything over-the-counter or alternative medicines?
- Have any medications been changed recently?
- Are you allergic to anything that you know of?

FHx

- Do any conditions run in the family? Consider asking specifics as for PMHx!
- Has anyone in the family ever had any skin yellowing like this?

SHx

- Smoking/ Alcohol (Hepatitis/ Cirrhosis)/ Recreational drugs (IVDU Hepatitis!)
  - ➢ Ask about tattoos/ blood transfusions/ acupuncture
- Home environment? Have you been getting support to cope with everything?
- Occupation – What do you do for a living if you don't mind me asking? How has this impacted on your life and occupation?

Summarise and Thank

- I'd just like to summarise back to you to make sure I haven't missed anything
- Is there anything you'd like to talk about that we haven't quite addressed?
- Thank you for talking to me and I wish you all the best

Investigations

Examination	Abdominal examination
Bedside	Urine dip
Bloods	FBC, cell counts, LDH, haptoglobin, LFTs, clotting, tumour markers, hepatitis serology.
Imaging	USS abdomen, CT CAP
Special	Blood films for spherocytosis, and genetic testing (Wilson's, haemochromatosis etc.)

Differential Diagnosis

	Diagnosis	Features In History	Features In Investigations	Management
PRE-HEPATIC	**Haemolysis**	Anaemia: lethargy, SOBOE, pallor. May have history of malaria / mechanical heart valve / new medications. May have abdominal pain from gallstones if long term. Dark urine and pale stools. TTP: fever and neuro symptoms. FH / personal Hx: spherocytosis, G6PD deficiency, sickle cell.	Exam: pallor, tachycardia. May have splenomegaly in red cell disorders. Bloods: anaemia, raised bilirubin, haptoglobin and LDH. Raised reticulocyte count. Schistocytes on blood film. Deranged U&E if TTP.	Management of underlying cause – stop medication / treat trigger. Prophylactic folate for red cell synthesis and avoiding megaloblastosis. Transfusion if Hb <70. Haematology referral.
HEPATIC	**Viral Hepatitis**	RUQ pain, fever, jaundice, malaise and return from endemic country for Hepatitis A – faeco-oral risk factors (street food, non-filtered water). Hepatitis B – travel to endemic areas. Preceded by vomiting and fever.	Exam: jaundice, dehydration from vomiting. Bloods: abnormal LFTs, raised bilirubin. Positive serology for viral hepatitis.	Acute Hep A & B: Self-limiting, supportive treatment. Chronic Hep B: Antivirals, monitor for HCC. Hep C: interferon therapy in acute and antivirals in chronic.
	Hepatocellular carcinoma	Jaundice, RUQ fullness, maybe ascites. B-symptoms. History of Hep B/C, Aclohol excess, haemochromatosis, NASH	Exam: RUQ fullness, hepatomegaly. Bloods: AFP raised, abnormal LFTs and coagulation. CT: liver mass.	MDT. Surgical resection and liver transplant is usually the best outcome.
	Also Consider: Drugs like paracetamol/ penicillins (e.g. co-amoxiclav) that can cause cholestasis			
POST-HEPATIC	**Gall stones**	History of intermittent RUQ pain, especially after fatty meal, associated nausea, may be colicky (biliary colic), jaundice. Likely had similar pains before, self-resolving. RFs: "4 Fs" fat, female, forties, fertile	Murphy's positive on examination, guarding. Raised WCC and CRP, abnormal LFTs (obstructive pattern, raised ALP and GGT) USS shows cholecystitis or cholelithiasis	Antibiotics (ceftriaxone and Metronidazole) and planned cholecystectomy in 4-6 weeks if stable.
	Cancer at head of pancreas	Painless jaundice, b-symptoms. history of pancreatitis, recent new DM, pruritus.	Exam: RUQ mass, non-tender with jaundice. Bloods: obstructive LFTS (raised GGT and ALP > AST and ALT). Raised amylase and lipase. Raised CA 19-9, CEA.	MDT approach for management. Notorious for late diagnosis and poor prognosis. Surgical: Whipple's procedure. Chemotherapy

Marking Criteria JAUNDICE	Marks	
	Awarded	Available
Washed hands at the start of the station		1
Introduced themselves – Including First name, last name and role		1
Patient details confirmed: Full name, Age/ D.O.B.		1
Explained purpose of consultation		1
Open question about what brings the patient in today + Clarification of any ambiguity		1

Timeline allows a clear understanding of onset and progression
   - Onset/ Circumstance
   - Sudden vs. gradual
   - Fluctuations
   - Progression
   - Past episodes
		3

Symptoms elicited are relevant and clearly directed at either arriving at a diagnosis or excluding other plausible diagnoses
   - Itching
   - Confusion
   - Recent viral illness
   - General enquiry – other than the yellowing, have you noticed any other changes?
		5

Systems queried are relevant to the complaint and adequate questions are asked for each symptom - Gastrointestinal; Genitourinary; Constitutional; **RECENT TRAVEL**; **SEXUAL CONTACT**		5
Explores **Ideas, Concerns and Expectations**		3
Elicits relevant **Past Medical History** - Autoimmune disease; Gallstones; Hepatitis; Cirrhosis; Cancer		2
Elicits relevant **Drug History** including **Allergies**		2
Elicits relevant **Family History**		2
Elicits relevant **Social History** – including Smoking/ alcohol/ recreational drugs + Tattoos/ Transfusions/ Acupuncture; **H**ome environment & support; **O**ccupation & impact on life		2
Closes consultation appropriately allowing the patient to ask any questions		1
Presentation: structured, concise		2
Appropriate Differential Diagnosis ± Investigations ± Management Plan		3
Examiner mark – professionalism and rapport		5
Patient mark – professionalism and rapport		5

Consultation	Presentation	Global marks patient	Global marks examiner	Total
‾‾30‾‾	‾‾5‾‾	‾‾5‾‾	‾‾5‾‾	‾‾45‾‾

17M presenting to hospital with acute jaundice

HPC	Patient presents with 2-weeks history of general malaise and feeling unwell. He reports some nausea, vomiting, fever and abdominal pain. 2 days ago, he noticed that his eyes were turning yellow and has now discovered that his skin is also turning yellow. He feels like his abdomen is more distended and particularly painful on the right side. He also states that he has lost his appetite. He says he has recently travelled to Egypt with his family and spent some time in the rural areas of the Saini. He does not report any dizziness or headaches. He denies any contact with insects or needle stick injuries. No sexual contact.
PMHx	Appendectomy at age 7.
DHx	Nil regular.
SHx	No IVDU, no alcohol. No smoking. Lives with parents. Single.
FHx	Nil.
ICE	"I'm concerned that I have HIV/cancer"
Ix	FBC, U&E, LFT, coagulation screen, USS liver, stool sample, hepatitis viral screen, HIV test.
Dx	Viral Hepatitis (likely hepatitis A). Other less likely possibilities cholangitis, schistosomiasis
Tx	Supportive with IVI. Monitor liver function with regular LFTs. Pain relief as appropriate. Praziquantel if schistosomiasis

55M presents with acute abdominal pain and jaundice

HPC	Sudden onset severe abdominal pain. This is significantly worse in the upper half of the abdomen and feels worse on pressing on the left side of the abdomen. He feels dizzy, cold and feels that his heart is racing. He reports no trauma, LOC, CP but has noticed nausea and vomiting. He has not been eating in a while but reports that prior to this severe abdominal pain he had abdominal pain/fullness after meals. Patient reports feeling more comfortable when he leans forward.
PMHx	Previous admissions with abdominal pain, he absconded within 24 hours. Not registered with GP.
DHx	Patient says he takes daily ibuprofen for his bad knees. NKDA
SHx	Lives alone in council flat. Smokes 20 a day. Drinks 10 pints per day at least.
ICE	"Am I going to die?"
Ix	FBC, CRP, U&E, LFT, coagulation screen, Amylase, Vitamin B levels, erect chest x-ray to rule out perforation, USS Abdomen or CT abdomen if concerns of abdominal collection/ pseudocyst
Dx	Acute pancreatitis secondary to gallstones.
Tx	IV fluids, Alcohol detox medication, vitamin B compound/ Pabrinex, analgesia, consider cholecystectomy when stable. May need ITU support. Give alcohol cessation advice and refer to community alcohol nurse if patient gives consent.

22M presents with jaundice

HPC	Patient presents to hospital with 1-week history of yellowish discoloration of eyes which is getting darker. He says he thought it was related to a long night out with heavy drinking. Feels sick but reports no abdominal pain, palpitations, nausea or vomiting. No foreign travel. No SOB. No exposure to insects. He has not noticed any rash, joint pain/swelling and denies fever. He has been taking a lot of paracetamol recently as he has been in a lot of pain after going to the gym every day. Normally fit and healthy. Increased muscle bulk.
PMHx	Nil.
DHx	2g Paracetamol per day, NKDA.
SHx	Works as a personal trainer, watches his diet and health. Lives alone, no permanent partner. Denies use of IVDU or other illicit drugs. Has used "bulk up" pills a friend gave him
FHx	Dad diagnosed with liver cancer, currently on waiting list for transplant.
ICE	"Do you think I have liver cancer"
Ix	FBC, U&E, CRP, LFT, coagulation profile, in particular platelets, paracetamol levels, hepatitis serology, USS liver, liver biopsy, consider CT abdomen/pelvis
Dx	Drug induced (paracetamol) liver toxicity
Tx	Supportive. Monitoring. NAC, referral to the liver unit if LFT/INR continue to worsen – Read up King's College Hospital Liver Transplant Criteria.

WORK WITH UNIADMISSIONS

UniAdmissions is the UK's number one university admissions company, specialising in **supporting applications to Medical School and to Oxbridge**. Every year, *we* help thousands of applicants and schools across the UK. From free resources to these *Ultimate Guide Books* and from intensive courses to bespoke individual tuition, *UniAdmissions* boasts a team of **500 Expert Tutors** and a proven track record of producing great results.

UniAdmissions is always looking for enthusiastic tutors to help nurture tomorrow's talent. In addition to gaining valuable teaching and training skills, tutoring with us allows you to gain vital application points for your core medical or surgical training applications. All our medical tutors have the option of completing free teaching and training courses to help give their medical/surgical applications a much needed boost and stand out from the crowd.

In addition, you're guaranteed to earn more than £ 100 per day's work; to find out more visit: **www.uniadmissions.co.uk/work-with-us**

YOUR FREE FPAS SJT BOOK

Thanks for purchasing this Ultimate Guide Book. Readers like you have the power to make or break a book – hopefully you found this one useful and informative. If you have time, *UniAdmissions* would love to hear about your experiences with this book.

As thanks for your time we'll send you a copy of our *Ultimate SJT Guide: 300 Practice Questions* absolutely <u>FREE</u>!

How to Redeem Your Free Ebook in 3 Easy Steps
1) Find the book you have either on your Amazon purchase history or your email receipt to help find the book on Amazon.
2) On the product page at the Customer Reviews area, click on 'Write a customer review'
Write your review and post it! Copy the review page or take a screen shot of the review you have left.

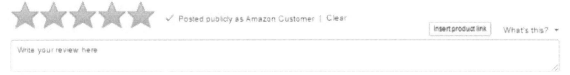

3) Head over to **www.uniadmissions.co.uk/free-book** and select the FPAS SJT book.

Your ebook will then be emailed to you – it's as simple as that!

Alternatively, you can buy this at **www.uniadmisions.co.uk/our-books**

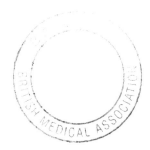

Printed in Poland
by Amazon Fulfillment
Poland Sp. z o.o., Wrocław